Dental Team Companion

Dental Team Companion

By

**Carole Brennan
Jenny Gallagher
Marina Harris
Michael Martin
Gail Vernon
Nairn Wilson
Liana Zoitopoulos**

Editor-in-Chief: Nairn H F Wilson
Editor: Mabel Slater

Quintessence Publishing Co. Ltd.
London, Berlin, Chicago, Paris, Milan, Barcelona, Istanbul,
São Paulo, Tokyo, New Delhi, Moscow, Prague, Warsaw

British Library Cataloguing in Publication Data

Dental team companion. – (Quintessentials of dental practice)
1. Dental teams.
I. Series II. Brennan, Carole.
617.6'023–dc22

ISBN-13: 9781850971214

Copyright © 2009 Quintessence Publishing Co. Ltd., London

Illustrators: Elizabeth and Paul Ducker

ISBN-13: 978-1-85097-121-4

Foreword

The dental team approach is the future of oral healthcare provision. As with any team, members must have shared goals, together with a clear understanding of the roles and responsibilities of each member. In addition, to be effective, a team must react and deal with situations as a team rather than as a group of individuals. This companion promotes the adoption of the team approach considered necessary for success in modern oral healthcare provision.

Putting the patient first in a patient-centred approach to the provision of oral healthcare is critical to the success of a dental team. To meet the needs and expectations of the patient, with favourable clinical outcomes, requires a concerted team approach to achieve continuing quality improvement in the quest for excellence. Success in this venture, as set out in this thought-provoking addition to the nearly complete highly acclaimed Quintessentials of Dental Practice Series, requires an understanding by the dental team of patients' attitudes in our ever-changing society, the culture and dynamics of the workplace and the many, varied facets of contemporary professionalism.

As with all the other volumes in the Quintessential of Dental Practice Series, this companion is intended to be read in a few hours and to have an immediate impact on the reader's approach to clinical practice. The dental team approach has many advantages and benefits, but these can only be realised through strong professional team working focused on doing the very best for each and every patient in a safe, confidence-inspiring practice environment – the thrust of this book.

To some, this Quintessentials volume may be a revelation; to others, it may provide reassurance that their dental team has the right approach to success. Whatever is taken from this book, it can only enhance benefits to patients and dental professionalism.

Nairn Wilson
Editor-in-Chief

Preface

Since the mid 1990s, there have been major changes to almost every aspect of dentistry. Scientific contributions to clinical and laboratory practice have resulted in dramatic advances. Together with a move to evidence-based practice, we can now offer our patients an ever-increasing range of choices as to their treatment options.

The ethos of dentistry has changed and everyone has now signed up to the concept of teamwork, offering the optimum dental care. Dentists nowadays no longer consider working single-handedly. Indeed, the vast majority could not work without the support of a wide range of dental care professionals.

This book gives all members of the dental team the chance to explore how their roles have developed and to gain insight into the opportunities that are emerging to further extend their working practices. These innovations will offer improved patient care and help to enhance the day-to-day working lives of the dental team.

There are three main chapter groups within this book. The first chapters look at how we continue to put the patient first, both in the context of the wider society and also within the clinical setting. Offering understanding and respect to our patients, let alone other members of the dental team, helps us to realise the importance of the good communication practices that are essential for all interactions with our patients and colleagues. Sometimes things may go wrong. It is important that we recognise this and our role in handling patient's complaints, hopefully with positive outcomes.

The second group of chapters deals with the culture of the workplace, encouraging us to look at ourselves in our day-to-day working environment. Sometimes we lack the opportunity to take time out of our busy working lives to reflect on how we can develop and improve our approach to work. This group of chapters will hopefully stimulate our thought processes and enable us to avoid conflict, reduce stress and, when all else fails, reflect on how to make things better.

The final chapters concentrate on professionalism and, as members of the dental team, how we can recognise the importance of maintaining high standards both at work and in our personal lives. Continuing professional and personal development allows us to keep up to date in a rapidly changing working environment. We can no longer be expected to retain all the information we gained during our professional education and training, and as ideas, materials and working practices move forward, we need to keep up to date actively.

This book has been designed to give an overview of team working for all dental team members. It aims to contribute to the core skills and understanding required of oral healthcare professionals in today's world.

This Quintessentials volume should also be beneficial to all those considering returning to work after a career break. The book may be read from cover to cover or dipped into to read and learn about areas of special interest. It should stimulate further reading and associated personal development.

All members of the dental team will be aware that changes to legislation can affect their working livee. The roles and responsibilities of the members of the dental team are, in many countries, quite fluid. This book gives you an outline of current arrangements, although these may be subject to change. Being alert to such changes is important to you and your patients.

Enjoy this book and continue to enjoy the work that you do in the knowledge that you are making a great contribution to the dental care of your patients and, in turn, their quality of life.

Mabel Slater

Contents

Chapter 1
Putting the patient first
Changing society: moving with the times

Jenny Gallagher

Aim

The aim of this chapter is to outline how and why society is changing, examine trends in oral health and discuss the implications of both for contemporary healthcare and health professionals.

Outcome

Having read this chapter, readers should have a greater understanding of the challenges of providing healthcare in modern society and have considered how oral healthcare professionals should respond to changing times.

Introduction

The world is in a period of intense change. Those in contemporary industrial societies are surrounded by a myriad of 'choices', which can be bewildering. We are bombarded with advertising about the latest fashions, food and lifestyle accompaniments so that we can keep up to date in terms of what we wear, do, think and act. Whatever our background, our lifestyles are very different from those of our parents, let alone our grandparents. There are greater opportunities for making and keeping contact with others through modern telecommunications, yet more people than ever live on their own, disconnected from their family networks. Thus paradoxically at one level, the world seems more 'connected' through the internet and population movement, but at another level is can be fragmented and lonely. Change is one of the constants of modern-day living.

Changing society

The values of society
Sociologists comment on the changes in the structure and nature of society and its values. The values important for guiding us through the complexity of life are strongly influenced by the prevailing culture. The 'wants' of

1

individuals are constantly escalating, driven by advertising and what others have. Consequently, we find ourselves living in an increasingly 'individualistic' and 'commercialised' society.

Sociologists suggest that we have never had it so good or lived so long; however, major inequalities exist. One of the impacts of these changes is that we are faced with a range of choices and we have to make many, varied decisions about our lifestyle. Therefore, developing personal values is very important to help navigate life in present-day society.

Health professionals complain that they are increasingly bombarded with information and choice. There are pressures to use new materials, develop new skills and adopt new techniques and systems as they endeavour to keep up to date professionally. Patients are becoming more knowledgeable. Both patients and health systems are becoming more demanding and health professionals are required to be more accountable for what they do. Workforce roles in the dental team are expanding and health systems are reforming around the world. Standing back and reflecting on society can help the healthcare professional to manage the daily challenges of professional life

This chapter draws on public health and behavioral and social sciences, which includes the study of society and how it functions, and the study of behavior and experience. The implications for healthcare are examined in the course of the chapter. Finally, it examines how we as health professionals should respond to changing times.

Demography

The population of high-income countries has changed dramatically over the past 100 or so years; overall the birth rate has reduced but people are living longer and the population is growing in size. A very clear visual demonstration of this dramatic change in the UK population is shown in Fig 1-1. As shown in Fig 1-2, the rate of change is set to increase and population growth is anticipated to increase more rapidly than expected because of longevity, rising immigration and higher birth rates amongst immigrant families. Assessments of social diversity, based on social class, income and education, suggest that the gap between the most affluent and the poorest in society is increasing. Furthermore, societies are becoming more multicultural, a fact that is very apparent in many large urban areas, but is not exclusive to such areas. Hence, populations are increasingly characterised by age and ethnic diversity. If a dental practice is located in an area in which there are a lot of young people, then it is likely that the patient base will involve many families. Dental practices in areas where people retire will have many older people as patients. If this link between the patient demographics and the local demographics is not apparent, then the dental team may wish to consider if it is serving the local community and whether changes are necessary to enable it to do so. Each section of the community will have particular oral health needs and expectations, cultural needs in the way care is provided and different barriers to accessing care.

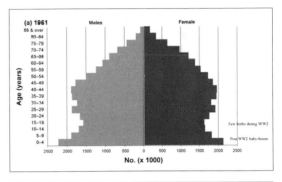

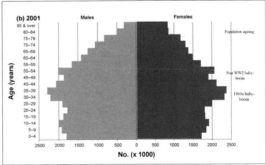

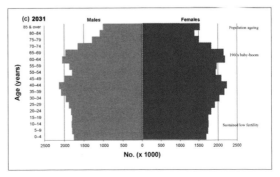

Fig 1-1 UK Population structure by age and sex in (a) 1951, (b) 2001 and (c) as predicted in 2031. WW2, World War II. (Adapted from the Office for National Statistics, Census 1951 and Census 2001.)

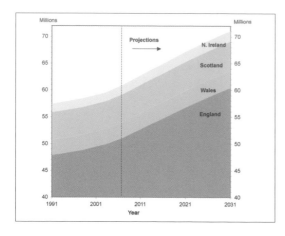

Fig 1-2 National populations in the countries of the UK. Population of the UK is projected to rise to 71 million by 2031. (Reproduced from the Office for National Statistics, 2007.)

Trends in health and illness

In high-income countries, disease patterns and mortality rates have changed. This is associated with improvements in living conditions and healthcare. Together with these changes, there has been a reduction in acute conditions, but an increase in chronic health problems. Death in childhood is now uncommon compared with a century ago. Most people will live into old age and, over time, develop a range of chronic conditions that will require specific management. Internationally, the key general health challenges are associated with cardiovascular disease, cancers, mental and sexual health problems and conditions such as diabetes. However, marked inequalities in health exist according to social, ethnic and sexual demography within and between countries across the world.

Trends in oral health

Patterns of oral health change over time. They also vary between and within countries, as well as across age groups and social groups. In the UK, as in a number of other countries, national oral health surveys play an important role in monitoring oral diseases and conditions. They also examine reported health behaviours and expectations of the population. The data are collected through clinical epidemiological surveys of a random sample of children and adults, plus associated questionnaires or interview. The information from such surveys is important to inform practice and policy relating to dentistry. The broad trends in oral and dental diseases and conditions are examined below. These highlight the different patterns of care required for children and young people, adults and older individuals. Of all the oral conditions addressed by the dental team, dental caries, and its long-term effects, remains the most common. As people live longer, and retain more of their teeth, they have an increased risk of developing caries, together with all the related conditions from gum diseases to toothwear, at some stage in their remaining life.

Impact of oral conditions

Approximately one in five children and one in two adults in industrialized countries report that their oral health impacts on their daily living. Pain and psychological impacts are most common, with a small proportion of adults feeling handicapped and unable to cope with their condition. This demonstrates the importance of good oral health and healthcare for general well-being.

Attitudes to oral health and accessing dental care

Overall, the UK population has positive attitudes towards oral and dental health, as demonstrated by, for example, the desire to retain teeth into old age, parents taking their children for oral healthcare and more regular dental attendance amongst middle-aged adults. It is also reflected in the increasing use of oral hygiene products. Barriers to dental care are well recognised to be fear, cost, fear of cost, lack of perception of need and features of the dental surgery. The latter includes how patients are managed at reception, waiting times and the personalities of the dental professionals. All of these factors can be reduced by good communication skills and patient-centred care.

Dental caries

Recent decades have seen significant reductions in the level of dental caries in high-income populations. Until relatively recently, having tooth decay in such populations was accepted as a fact of life and few adults had not experienced tooth decay or tooth loss. Denture wearing in middle-aged and older people was common. Another change is the pattern of tooth decay; whereas in the past many restorations involved the mesial, occlusal and distal surfaces, perhaps with buccal and lingual extensions, now, they are most likely to affect only the occlusal surface. These changes are largely attributed to fluoride in toothpaste (used by the majority) and, where available, fluoridated water.

Despite improvements in oral health, many children continue to experience tooth decay. Few other diseases are as common in children and young people and it is particularly amongst those living in social deprivation. Improvements

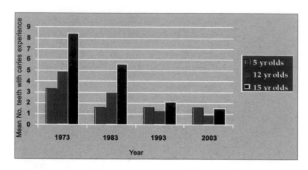

Fig 1-3 Trends in average levels of caries in children. Average number of missing and filled teeth by age in children in England and Wales 1973–1993 and in the UK in 2003. (Data from UK Child Dental Health Surveys: O'Brian (1994), Pitts and Harker (2004).)

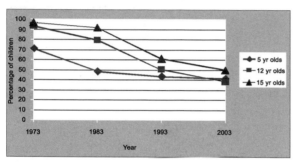

Fig 1-4 Trends in prevalence of dental caries in children. Percentage of children with decay experience in England and Wales 1973–1993 and in the UK in 2003. (Data from UK Child Dental Health Surveys: O'Brian (1994), Pitts and Harker (2004).)

in oral health tend to have slowed and have reached a plateau in young children (Figs 1-3 and 1-4). Further improvements will require a greater emphasis on health promotion and prevention.

Amongst adults in most countries, there are growing expectations of retaining a functioning dentition into old age, preferably without recourse to dentures. Overall, fewer teeth are being extracted; however, most adults are locked into the restorative cycle and require more complex dentistry as the size and complexity of replacement restorations increase. Middle-aged and older people are well placed to understand the risks of oral disease and, with the desire to retain their teeth, may be highly motivated to adopt preventive approaches to their dental care. Older people, 55 years of age and over, are prone to chronic health conditions. Medication may increase the risk of oral disease in association with reduced salivary flow and changes in diet.

Periodontal diseases
Periodontal diseases affect the majority of the population to some extent. The more severe forms of periodontal diseases, which may be the principal cause of tooth loss, only occur in a minority (5–15%). There is some evidence

that periodontal diseases are related to age and social status. The disease is cumulative and, therefore, as more people retain their natural teeth, more are at risk of periodontal diseases. National surveys show that the level and severity of disease rises with increasing age.

Toothwear

As teeth remain in the oral cavity for longer, they are at risk of toothwear. Toothwear is a natural consequence of ageing and will increasingly be a problem in older people who retain their natural teeth. There is some worrying evidence that this type of wear is increasing in young people, with one third of 15 year olds having tooth surface loss on their incisors lingually and 4% having dentine or pulp exposure on their first permanent molars (Chadwick and Pendry, 2004). This is associated with a range of intrinsic factors, such as bulimia or gastric reflux, and extrinsic factors, such as the consumption of large quantities of acidic and carbonated drinks.

Oral cancer

Oral cancer is the most serious of the oral conditions likely to present in a dental surgery. The risk of developing oral cancer increases with age. It is strongly related to social and economic deprivation, with the highest rates occurring in the most disadvantaged sections of the population. Risk factors include smoking and excessive consumption of alcohol, particularly when combined, and low intake of vitamins. Preventive advice and support are important for people with these risk behaviours.

Current challenges

Oral health in many countries has never been better; however, major inequalities persist. There are wide variations in oral health across age groups and geographically and socially. Much of the impact of dental caries is seen in middle-aged and older people, who will have expectations of retaining their dentition while at risk of restorative failure, periodontal diseases and toothwear. Many of the preventive and reparative procedures in children and young adults with relatively good oral health are increasingly simple. Challenges for dental teams, therefore, relate to the dental care of middle-aged and older people and vulnerable groups, who require holistic care including skillful management of their medical and social challenges.

A major challenge is the need to convert irregular attendees to regular users of primary dental care services.

Healthcare in a changing society

Globalisation

Globalisation is the growing interdependence between different peoples, regions and countries. The effects of globalisation are seen in the worldwide sale of specific products such as Coca-Cola, which can be found on a remote African roadside stall and in an American superstore. It is seen in the manufacture of goods such as cars, where individual components will be manufactured in different countries and continents and then transported and assembled in another country to produce an 'international product'. People increasingly move around the world in search of jobs and opportunities, bringing with them their culture and diversity. All of these changes are breaking down traditional ways of doing things, thus presenting individuals with the challenge of creating and recreating self-identities.

Patient-centred healthcare

The relationship between health professionals and patients has changed dramatically over recent decades. Societies are moving away from a paternalistic approach, where the healthcare professional knows best and is in charge, to one in which the patient is centre stage. As a result, there is an increasing emphasis on involving patients in treatment planning decisions and the public in fashioning health policy.

At the individual level, empowerment of patients is demonstrated by making it easy for patients to have appointments of their choice, discussing care options and plans, seeking informed consent and allowing choice over referral to specialist or hospital care. Empowerment of patients, therefore, includes choices, rights and participation in decision making about their health and healthcare. This is especially important in dentistry, where adult patients are typically required to pay for some or all of their treatment and are, therefore, consumers as well as patients.

> Empowerment of patients includes choice, rights and participation in decision making.

The internet explosion has had a major impact on healthcare. It facilitates self-diagnosis and self-treatment at home. Furthermore, the chronic nature of most health problems means that the patient readily becomes expert in relation to his/her condition. Patient support groups for particular conditions contribute to this process, further changing the patient–professional relationship.

Healthcare delivery

There is increasing awareness that wider issues, such as how, when, where and by whom care is delivered, are just as important as what care is delivered. Governments look at it in terms of providing quality, access and choice, or value for money. However, many aspects are judged in terms of process as well as outcomes.

Where care is delivered

Contemporary influences mean that there is greater emphasis on self-care, moving care out of hospitals, and developing outreach services for vulnerable groups. At one end of the spectrum, it is recognised that care is provided in all settings from home to hospital. Promoting self-care, in particular preventive care, is really important in support of a healthy society. Analysts suggest that to optimise the health of the population, let alone achieve the most cost-effective care, people need to be fully engaged with their health.

In contrast to medicine, in which a large part of care has traditionally been in hospitals, the majority of dental care has always been provided in a primary care setting. However, to achieve equity of access and outcome, some vulnerable groups may require outreach services. This can take the form of mobile services for homeless people or providing domiciliary care for people who are housebound.

The funding of dental care

For many patients, cost and fear of cost are important barriers to dental care. This is why state-funded care, as provided by the National Heath Service (NHS) in the UK, is important in the provision of healthcare. One of the greatest political and professional challenges ahead is to ensure that the resources going into dental care are sufficient to meet public needs and are used to provide the greatest benefit possible. This should include funding for health promotion, including preventive care.

Cultural sensitivity

There are cultural and language barriers to the delivery of healthcare. An understanding of society can assist in providing culturally sensitive healthcare and so reduce barriers to dental care. Scully and Wilson (2006), in the *Quintessentials of Dental Practice* series, suggested that healthcare systems should be accessible with due regard to the beliefs, attitudes and cultural lifestyles of both the patient and the professional. This should include culture, race, gender, sexual orientation, social class and economic situation. Examples include sensitivity in treating women, who may prefer to be treated by a female member

9

of the team, and Muslim women who wear a full veil. In such circumstances, it is necessary to explore with patients what approach will be most acceptable to them, a principle that is helpful in the management of all patients.

Quality of care

There are several ways of looking at the quality of healthcare. Patients may judge healthcare with an emphasis on matters such as the welcome by, and empathy of the team, the general environment including the waiting room and the cost of care, rather than on the quality of a restoration.

There is increasing emphasis on ensuring that care has a sound scientific evidence base. Much of the care provided in dentistry is underpinned by traditional practice and professional opinion rather than being evidence-based. There are clear exceptions in the area of preventive dental care, where there is a significant body of well-researched knowledge that demonstrates the effectiveness of fluorides in protecting against dental caries.

In an attempt to improve quality, care is increasingly driven by clinical guidelines that are informed by the available evidence base, ideally using high quality evidence from systematic reviews and randomised controlled trials. This move is a direct response to spectacular failures by professionals and poor clinical outcomes. One good example is surgery for cleft lip and palate, where evaluation of the surgical outcomes in the UK showed that results were some of the worst in Europe. This led to the first dentally related set of national guidelines in the UK. The result was a gradual overhaul of the provision of care into a team approach underpinned by regular audit, resulting in greatly improved clinical outcomes. This approach is being increasingly used in respect to various aspects of oral healthcare across the world.

Delivering better oral health

Guidelines on evidence-based prevention have been published and are increasingly being adopted (Department of Health and British Association for the Study of Community Dentistry, 2007). Change is a slow process, but over time guidelines can influence society, as have initiatives to encourage the public to use oral hygiene products regularly.

Who delivers care?

Within healthcare generally there is increasing emphasis on team working. At the complex end of oral healthcare, this is demonstrated for head and neck cancer, where quality and outcomes frameworks have shown the importance of multidisciplinary teams providing care in an integrated manner. This may mean that patients will be under the care of several specialists, not just one specialist as tended to be the case in the past. There is also the view that complex care should be left to the experts. Dabbling in complex care is increasingly a thing of the past, so health professionals, including dental health professionals, have to consider whether cases are beyond their competence and expertise. Rare conditions need to be treated by experts and require patients to travel further for their care.

There is an expanding range of new healthcare professionals in medical and dental teams. Given the changing patterns of dental disease, much dental care is relatively routine in nature and may, according to national dental team provisions, be provided by, for example, dental therapists; this frees practitioners to provide complex care or care for patients with complex problems.

When care is delivered
Primary healthcare and, in particular, primary dental care have traditionally been provided on a Monday to Friday, 9–5 basis. Access to dental care has been a challenge for some time (Fig 1-5). In contemporary society, influenced by the consumer culture, there are increasing calls for better access to healthcare. People's working patterns, lack of job security and job

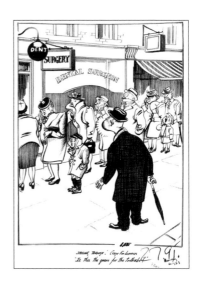

Fig 1-5 Queues are nothing new.... (Joseph Lee, 1943 Evening News (during World War II). Reproduced by permission of Solo Syndication / Associated Newspapers Ltd.)

11

inflexibility will mean that dental services will need to be provided for longer hours. This is entirely possible in line with providing job flexibility for members of the dental team, who, increasingly, have to juggle family and professional life. Furthermore, health policy increasingly places great importance on improving access to care, with reduced waiting times for first appointments and the start of treatment. Together they have implications for dental professionals' working hours.

Access to care
The public are increasingly accustomed to accessing care. However, some people in society who most need care do not access it on a regular basis; a small number never access dental care whilst others leave it so late that typically a tooth that could have been saved has to be extracted. Given inequalities in oral health across the social divide, it is of concern that the uptake of dental care is less frequent amongst people from socially deprived communities. There is clear evidence of inequalities in uptake of dental care at individual and population levels, even though in the UK those with low incomes do not have to pay for care. The common barriers to dental care have been well researched and the challenge for governments, policy makers and dental professionals is to minimise these barriers, notably fear, cost and fear of cost.

Access to oral health
Finally, it is important to recognise that gaining access to dental care is just one stage in a path to good oral health. This requires patients to understand their personal risks of oral disease and the measures that can be taken to reduce future risks. We live in a risk-averse culture and so society is likely to be more receptive to the potentials of prevention. Dental care professionals can play a vitally important role in promoting good diet, oral hygiene, use of fluoride and the uptake of clinical prevention such as fluoride varnishes and fissure sealants, as well as supporting patients in avoiding tobacco and misuse of alcohol.

Responding to the changing environment

If the dental team is to move with the times, serve its community and meet the ever increasing expectations of patients, it must reflect on its current structure, process and outcome on a regular basis. This can be assessed by asking a number of questions.

* What is the demography of the patient base?
* How does it relate to the local population?

- Do patients and the local community have specific dental or cultural needs?
- Are there particular groups who have poor access to dental care?
- Would any changes to the dental practice help to minimise barriers to dental care?
- How are patients' needs and demands explored?
- Is the care patient centred?
- Is care evidence based?
- What prevention is offered to patients?
- What use is made of skill mix in the dental team?

References

Chadwick B, Pendry L. Non-carious Dental Conditions: Children's Dental Health in the UK, 2003. London: Office for National Statistics, 2004.

Department of Health and the British Association for the Study of Community Dentistry. Delivering Better Oral Health: A Toolkit for Prevention. London: The Stationery Office, 2007. Available at: http://www.dh.gov.uk/en/Publicationsandstatistics/Publications/PublicationsPolicyAndGuidance/DH_078742.

O'Brian M. Children's Dental Health in the United Kingdom 1993. London: HMSO, 1994.

Office for National Statistics. Census 1951. London: Office of National Statistics. Available at: http://www.statistics.gov.uk.

Office for National Statistics. Census 2001. London: Office of National Statistics. Available at: http://www.statistics.gov.uk.

Pitts N, Harker R. Obvious decay experience: Children's dental health in the United Kingdom 2003. London: Office of National Statistics, 2004. Available at: http://www.statistics.gov.uk/children/dentalhealth/downloads/cdh_dentinal_decay.pdf.

Scully C, Wilson NHF. Culturally Sensitive Oral Healthcare. [Quintessentials of Dental Practice series, Vol. 35.] London: Quintessence, 2006.

Further reading

Cancer Research Council. UK Oral Cancer Incidence Statistics. London: Cancer Research Council, 2007. Available at: http://info.cancerresearchuk.org/cancerstats/types/oral/incidence/

Centre for Reviews and Dissemination:
http://www.york.ac.uk/inst/crd/crddatabases.htm

Cochrane Collaboration: http://www.cochrane.org/

Finch H, Keegan J, Ward K, Sanyal Sen B. Barriers to the Receipt of Dental Care: A Qualitative Study. London: Social and Community Planning Research, 1988.

Giddens A. Sociology, 5th edn. Cambridge: Polity Press, 2006.

Kelly M, Steele J, Nuttall N Bradnock G, Morris J., Nunn J, et al. Adult Dental Health Survey: Oral Health in the UK, 1998. London: The Stationery Office, 2000. Available at: http://www.statistics.gov.uk/STATBASE/Product.asp?vlnk=8112

Lader D, Chadwick B, Chestnutt I, Harker R, Morris J, Nuttall N, et al. Children's Dental Health in the UK. Summary Report for the Office for National Statistics, 2003. London: Office for National Statistics, 2005. Available at: http://www.statistics.gov.uk/STATBASE/Product.asp?vlnk=12918.

National Institute for Health and Clinical Excellence: http://www.nidcr.nih.gov/

Saltman RB, Figueras J, Sakellarides C (eds). Critical Challenges Facing Healthcare in Europe. Maidenhead, UK: Open University Press/McGraw-Hill Education for the European Observatory on Health Systems and Policies, 2000.

Chapter 2
Understanding and respect: caring for patients with special needs

Liana Zoitopoulos

Aim

The aim of this chapter is to explain the meaning of the term special needs and to address the special considerations required and issues raised when caring for patients with special needs.

Outcome

The chapter should lead to an understanding of what is meant by the term patients with special needs, and the importance of respecting each patient's individuality while taking into account the whole team that cares for such patients.

> The mark of a civilised society is the way it treats its disabled people.

Introduction

Definitions
Disability is defined as 'an anatomical, physiological or psychological loss or reduction in functional ability'. Impairment is defined as 'a disadvantage or restriction of activity due to a disability'.

The term special needs is commonly used to describe people who, because of a disability, are unable to perform some, many or all of the functions of everyday living. The terms special needs, disability, impairment and special care are all used to describe people who for a variety of reasons are in need of additional care. These terms will be used throughout this chapter.

Changing views of people with disability and special needs through time
Society has viewed disabled people in very different ways over the centuries. For example, babies born with disabilities in ancient Sparta were deemed

potentially unfit to live. Legend has it that they were left exposed on the inhospitable slopes of Mount Taygetos and only collected and taken home if they survived the night. Other sources say that they may have been thrown off a cliff. This attitude to those with impaired function seems to have been common in ancient times, although equally there are examples of people with disability achieving high office even then. In more recent times, the Victorians constructed buildings and transport systems that were impossible to access or use by many physically disabled people. Although lunatic asylums provided asylum for the mentally ill, there was also a perception that such institutions were required to separate those with mental illness from the community.

Often, the general population is ignorant about disability. People do not know how to behave and what is required of them when they are in the company of disabled persons. This is perhaps a reason why disabled people have tended to be excluded and isolated from mainstream general activities. They have also tended to be stigmatised. For example, in many cultures it remains difficult for parents to talk about having a disabled child. These are some of the reasons why disabled people have been placed in closed institutions, making integration with the rest of society difficult, if not impossible. There are many such examples even today. In parts of Europe, disabled children have been abandoned in institutions with very little care and no education whatsoever. Some countries still isolate people if they are infected with the human immunodeficiency virus (HIV) or have mental incapacity or illness. This has typically resulted in isolation and loss of dignity.

In the UK, even as recently as the late 20th century, society has tended to isolate disabled people, including those with mental illness. Disabled people were made dependent and institutionalised and to some extent this is still true. This approach, however, began to change towards the end of the last century when the move towards integration and empowerment of disabled people was initiated.

Of course, the creation of disabled entrances for buildings, although seemingly enabling inclusion, reinforces the impression that disabled people require special measures. More enlightened countries have placed a legal duty on those constructing public buildings to make them readily accessible to all through common entrances. Essentially, we have to decide whether the able-bodied and the disabled are two separate groups or part of the spectrum of humanity. The latter view, that those with disability are entitled to equal treatment, has been aided in the UK by the following legislation.

Disability Discrimination Act 1995

A person has a disability for the purposes of the Disability Discrimination Act if s/he has a physical or mental impairment which has a substantial and long-term adverse effect on his/her ability to carry out normal day-to-day activities. The Disability Discrimination Act 1995 requires that providers must:

* take reasonable steps to change policies, practices and procedures which make it unreasonably difficult or impossible for disabled people to use their services
* take reasonable steps to remove or alter physical features which could be a barrier to disabled people using their services
* provide the service in an alternative way if the removal of such barriers is impossible
* consider access to a service in broad terms that includes access to information about a service (e.g. information available as audio, large print and so on).

Disability Discrimination Act 2006

The 2006 modification of the original Disability Discrimination Act was designed to extend the rights for disabled people. It provided protection against discrimination for people using public services and it created new legal responsibilities for local authorities, agencies and other public bodies.

Mental Capacity Act 2005

The Mental Capacity Act, which came into full operation in October 2007, aims to protect people who cannot make decisions for themselves because of a learning disability, mental health condition or any other reason. It provides clear guidelines for carers and professionals about who can take decisions in which situations.

The Mental Capacity Act intends to protect people who lose the capacity to make their own decisions. It will:

* allow anyone, while they are still able, to appoint someone (e.g. a trusted relative or friend) to make decisions on their behalf in the event that they lose the ability to do so; the nominated individual can make decisions on the person's health and personal welfare where previously such an appointment only covered financial matters
* ensure that decisions that are made on the person's behalf are in their best interests and it provides a checklist of things that decision makers must work through

- introduce a code of practice for people such as healthcare workers who support people who have lost the capacity to make their own decisions.

The above changes in attitude and legislation have made at least the UK a far better place for disabled people. There is, however, still a long way to go.

Provision of oral care for disabled people

The branch of dentistry which tends to deal with the majority of disabled patients is known as special care dentistry (SCD). Its role has been defined in the UK by the Joint Advisory Committee for Special Care Dentistry as 'the improvement of oral health of individuals and groups in society who have a physical, sensory, intellectual, mental, medical, emotional or social impairment or disability or, more often, a combination of a number of these factors'.

SCD covers a diverse client group with a range of disabilities and complex additional needs. It must deal with people living at home, in long-stay residential care or in secure units, in addition to the homeless. It requires a holistic approach that is specialist led to meet the complex requirements of people with impairments.

During the journey from receiving a referral to providing oral care for a patient with special needs to completing their care, it must always be kept in mind that there are two distinct types of patient to consider. SCD provides simple dental care for patients with complex comorbidities, or complex dentistry for patients with more straightforward problems (Fig 2-1). Finally, some patients seen by the SCD team are in the transition period between paediatric and adult services, when it is easy for them to be lost in the system.

There are several types of impairment seen in the patient population dealt with by special care clinicians:

- physical disability
- medical disability
- intellectual disability
- mental illness
- sensory disability
- people who are anxious or phobic.

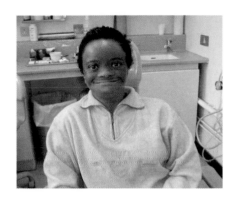

Fig 2-1 Intellectually impaired patient with simple dental needs.

Such individuals have special needs and their dental needs are no exception. The following text discusses these groupings in more detail.

Physical disability

There is a wide range of conditions which may lead to physical disability. Such disabilities are often congenital or develop relatively early in life. These might include patients with various inherited neuromuscular disorders (e.g. Duchenne muscular dystrophy, myotonic dystrophy or spinal muscular atrophy) or neuromuscular conditions acquired during childhood (e.g. poliomyelitis, which was once a serious problem). Brain injury around the time of birth may lead to severe physical impairment in the form of cerebral palsy. Traumatic injury to the spinal cord may also lead to profound physical impairment. In later life, cerebrovascular and musculoskeletal disease may lead to profound physical disability.

Patients with physical disability may well have preserved full intellectual function, and this must be remembered at all times.

Medical disability

Patients with medical disability are those who have chronic medical conditions that have a significant impact on day-to-day activities, or those whose condition requires the administration of long-term or complex medication. Many will present with dental disease that requires careful assessment and treatment, given their underlying condition (Fig 2-2). The dental treatment in itself may be straightforward. Such patients generally fall into the following broad categories of disease or disorder:

19

- congenital or acquired heart disease
- respiratory disorders such as cystic fibrosis, asthma, bronchitis
- immunosuppression as a result of disease or drugs
- diabetes, either insulin or non-insulin dependent
- bleeding disorders as a consequence of disease or drugs
- neurological disorders, such as Parkinson's disease, motor neurone disease, multiple sclerosis, Alzheimer's disease.

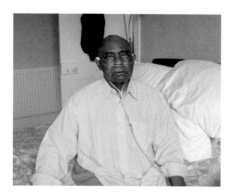

Fig 2-2 Domicillary visit to a patient with a complex medical history. His treatment was subsequently arranged in a hospital.

Intellectual disability

Patients with intellectual disability vary widely between those with mild impairment of intellectual function to those who require almost constant supervision. Underlying causes include Down's syndrome, cerebral palsy, congenital hypothyroidism, microcephaly, epilepsy or global developmental delay.

Mental illness

This may vary in severity from relatively minor difficulty in leading an apparently normal lifestyle to complete incapacity with dependence on others. The underlying causes include schizophrenia, bipolar disorder, post-traumatic stress disorder and depression.

Sensory disability

Sensory disability refers to deafness and blindness. There are a very large number of causes. These conditions may be present from birth or develop later in life.

Anxiety and phobias

Some patients suffer from anxieties or phobias. These include agoraphobia, claustrophobia and needle phobia. Patients with eating disorders, anorexia nervosa and bulimia, may present with dental problems.

Treatment issues

General considerations

There is a common thread running through many of these varied conditions associated with disability: the patient is, to a greater or lesser extent, dependent on a carer or carers in order to perform sometimes even the simplest function.

For example, a patient who has had a liver transplant is dependent on their liver specialist unit for monitoring of liver function and supervision of the large number of immunosuppressive drugs which must be taken. These provide a complex challenge to the dental team, and close liaison with the liver specialists is essential prior to considering dental treatment. A person with severe intellectual or physical impairment may be directly dependent on their carer for most functions of daily living. It goes without saying that any carers need to be closely involved in the provision of dental care. It is, therefore, important to emphasise that special considerations are required when such a patient needs dental care. These considerations are dependent on both the dental condition and the associated disability.

It is critical to successful treatment to recognise that not all disability is accompanied by intellectual impairment. Even if it is, there are gradations of intellectual impairment, ranging from mild through moderate to severe. In all cases of intellectual impairment, the dental team should attempt to have direct communication with the patient.

Patients who understand what is going on, but are dependent, often feel frustrated or embarrassed that they are being a nuisance to those around them. It is important to recognise this and make them feel appreciated and special. It is also worth acknowledging that, despite being dependent, patients are still in charge of their own destiny. Their carers should not try to govern what the patient should have done. Carers sometimes do this out of convenience for themselves and, at other times, because they think they know best. Once these fundamental issues have been addressed and understood, then, and only then, can the practicalities of caring for patients with special needs in the dental setting be addressed.

Dental considerations

By the very nature of the observations above, it is clear that the approach to SCD must be as a team: clinician, receptionist, nurse, hygienist and therapist. In turn, the dental team must work in conjunction with all the other healthcare professionals involved in the care of the disabled patient. These may include the doctor, the speech and language therapist, the psychiatrist and the district nurse. The dentist is the leader of the dental team and must ensure that good communication channels are in place.

The receptionist is a vital member of the team. This individual is generally the first point of contact with the patient or carer, and the one who makes the appointment and reminds the patient of it. They will also have the responsibility of ensuring that transport has been organised, once the clinician has confirmed the necessity for this.

The nurse is often the first clinical member of the dental team that disabled patients and their carers will come into contact with, since he or she will welcome the patient and bring them from the waiting area into the surgery. Often the patients will speak to the nurse rather than to the clinician, disclosing information that may make a major difference to their overall dental care.

The hygienist or the therapist forms an integral part of the team, since together with the clinician he or she will ensure that the patient's oral hygiene is kept to a high standard and dietary habits maintained or improved.

Consent

It is essential that informed consent is obtained for all treatment, although written consent is not always required. It should be emphasised that a signed form is not proof of informed consent.

When informed consent cannot be obtained, it is usually necessary with intellectually impaired patients to hold a best-interest meeting. This is a meeting between all those healthcare professionals involved in the care of the patient. The clinician sets out the dental management plan to render the patient dentally fit and asks the whole team to consider whether this is in the best interest of the patient. Once agreement has been reached, an informed decision involving all with knowledge of the patient's needs, then the clinician can proceed with the treatment plan.

> Informed consent is an essential prerequisite for treatment.

For all the above reasons, one of the most important factors in deciding how to manage the patient is time. Adequate time set aside for planning will ensure that the correct information has been gathered, and it will allow the patients to maintain their dignity.

Care of the patient in the surgery

Before the patient has arrived in the surgery, s/he will have already negotiated several hurdles. For example, if a patient is taking long-term medication they will have to have taken their medication prior to visiting the dental surgery.

It is essential to take a good medical history. The importance of this cannot be stressed enough. It is helpful to do this thoroughly in an unhurried manner, since taking time is a good way of creating a relationship with the patient. Allow the patient time to establish trust in the team. It is not always easy to discuss a disability and some patients take a long time before they do so.

The patient's social context is very important. It is first worth establishing whether the patient is living in an institution or at home. In either event, it should be noted who is caring for the patient, in particular whether it is the family or a carer, and if a carer whether they are permanent or transient. A transient carer may not know as much about the patient and this could affect the information gathering in relation to the patient's medical history. It is worth noting that double-checking may be necessary in this situation. Bear in mind, especially for patients with a learning disability, that information may have to be cross-referenced with that given by the doctor looking after the patient and with the carer.

People with disabilities often experience barriers to receiving care. These may be factors relating to their previous experience, such as rejection, lack of control and fear; environmental barriers, such as lack of wheelchair access or a lift; general caring facilities; transport and access; and availability of sources of advice. There may be barriers relating to healthcare professionals, such as cultural attitudes, lack of sympathy, personal beliefs and lack of training.

The medical history for every patient should be updated at each visit. Changes may occur from one week to the next that may have far-reaching consequences when treating a patient. For example, if a patient suffering from heart disease needs a dental extraction, it is possible that they may have been placed on warfarin therapy between visits, inhibiting blood clotting. Extractions under such circumstances will inevitably mean extreme difficulty, if not failure, in stopping bleeding from the socket.

It is essential to plan and prepare for treatment before the patient arrives. This will allow the patient to be greeted appropriately and allow full concentration on the patient from the moment they enter the surgery.

It is rude to talk over any patient as if they were not there, and those with intellectual impairment are no different. Although the carer will inevitably have additional information, questions should be addressed to the patient, and only indirectly to the carer. If the carer attempts to take over the consultation, as sometimes happens, the dental health professional must try to strike an appropriate balance.

In terms of initiating treatment, it is worth checking whether premedication is necessary and ensuring that there is time for this to take effect before treatment is started.

Domiciliary care
If a patient is not able to come to a surgery, then the surgery can, to an extent, be taken to the patients' home. This is known as a domiciliary service (Fig 2-3).

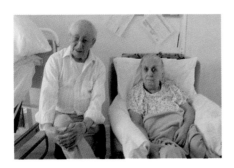

Fig 2-3 Domiciliary visit to a patient cared for by her husband.

The types of treatment which can be offered during a domiciliary visit include:

- assessment
- extractions
- dentures
- dressings
- simple fillings
- scale and polish
- assessment after a general anaesthetic.

In planning a domiciliary visit, the correct procedures for manual handling (e.g. transporting heavy equipment safely on a trolley) should be observed, as should the relevant infection control policies and procedures.

The following considerations should be borne in mind when preparing for a domiciliary visit.

- If there are to be a number of visits to different patients, it is helpful to group them geographically.
- The patient should be notified about the approximate time of arrival in advance, and it is also helpful to ring immediately before the visit as a reminder.
- While it may be tempting to try to transport the entire surgery, it is sensible to take only equipment that is likely to be used in order to minimise time and money spent (Fig 2-4).
- The patient's medical history should be checked before proceeding with treatment.
- At the end of the visit, all waste should be removed. The patient and carers should have relevant contact details in case of complications.

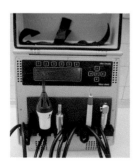 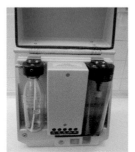 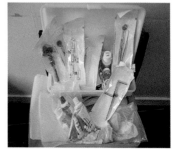

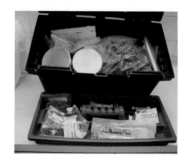

Fig 2-4 Equipment for a domiciliary visit.

There are advantages in trying to deliver care in the domiciliary setting. For the patient, they include improved access to dental care, increased independence, decreased fear of the unknown and greater autonomy. Advantages for the clinician include, most importantly, an opportunity to learn more about the patient, but also an opportunity to develop or improve skills such as time management and communication and liaison with other health workers. Domiciliary care is also potentially extremely rewarding professionally.

While it is impossible to cover all the conditions dealt with in the context of SCD, some important specific examples are given below.

Conditions requiring specific approaches
Multiple sclerosis
Multiple sclerosis is a chronic neurological disorder characterised by varying symptoms between patients and over the course of time. The symptoms are extremely variable in severity but generally include fatigue, unsteadiness, vertigo, double vision and depression. The important considerations for the dental team are problems of access, coping with stress and vertigo in the reclined position.

Parkinson's disease
Parkinson's disease is another neurological condition, generally affecting a slightly older patient population and characterised by muscle rigidity, difficulty in and slowness of movement, tremor, involuntary movements, low-volume monotone voice, drooling and impaired swallowing (Fig 2-5). For the dental team, it is important to recognise that the patients may have a fear of their potential for random movements coupled with a sense of embarrassment about these involuntary movements and drooling of saliva. The common problems dentally include management of oral hygiene and dentures. Parkinsonian symptoms can occur with some medication and so knowledge of a patient's medical history will help in dealing with these too.

Disabling heart disease
For patients suffering from heart disease, it is important to communicate with their general medical practitioner to be informed of any changes in their medication. For example, it would be essential to know if the patient is taking warfarin as this inhibits clotting. It is important to ascertain the presence or absence of structural lesions within the heart, as these may require special management. Valve replacement, previous bacterial endocarditis, complex cyanotic heart defects and reconstruction of the major vessels all constitute

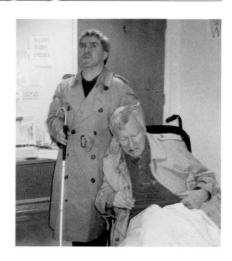

Fig 2-5 Patient suffering from Parkinson's disease, accompanied by his visually impaired partner.

a high risk for bacterial endocarditis after dental treatment and such patients should receive endocarditis prophylaxis before all dental procedures that involve bleeding.

Deafness
Deafness, whether it be mild, moderate, severe or profound, can cause difficulties in communication. People suffering from deafness are often concerned about the stigma associated with deafness. It is important to think about communication. Making sure that the patient can see the clinician's face is important if they rely on lip-reading.

Autism
Autism is characterised by difficulties in communication and social interaction, sensory overload and extreme discomfort with physical contact. This may lead to difficulties with access to the mouth in the dental surgery. Often the parent or carer can give useful advice on techniques to reduce the stress of treatment.

Alzheimer's disease
Alzheimer's disease is a dementing process characterised by, amongst other things, an insidious but slowly progressive onset of memory and judgement defects, changes in temperament, behavioural mood liability and personality change. The effects on carers include self-neglect, exhaustion, isolation and depression, often referred to as a 'living bereavement'. In the surgery, the

difficulties include inability to cope, particularly with communication, cooperation and concentration. Carers' fears in the dental situation relate to embarrassment, distress and the clinician's ability.

Conclusions

Disability has been viewed differently throughout the ages.

In the UK, the Disability Discrimination Acts and the Mental Capacity Act have improved the legal status of disabled people and their position within society.

The dental care of disabled people requires time and should be approached by the whole team.

Further reading

British Society for Oral Dentistry. Guidelines for Oral Health Care of People with Disabilities. Gosforth, UK: British Society for Oral Dentistry. Available at: www.bsdh.org.uk.

Department of Health. Valuing People's Oral Health: A Good Practice Guide for Improving the Oral Health of Disabled Children and Adults. London: The Stationery Office, 2007. Available at: www.dh.gov.uk/en/Publicationsandstatistics/Publications/PublicationsPolicyAndGuidance/DH_080918.

Fiske J, Dickinson C, Boyle C, Burke M. Special Care Dentistry. [Quintessentials series.] London: Quintessence, 2007.

Chapter 3
Patient interaction: engendering trust and confidence

Gail Vernon

Aim

The aim of this chapter is to encourage the dental team to be aware of the importance and implications of interaction with the patient.

Outcome

After reading this chapter, readers should have a greater understanding of how to ensure that the way they interact with patients is both positive and professional.

Introduction

Treat people as you would like to be treated

This maxim is central to effective patient interaction. You know how you like to be treated when you are the patient. You like to be treated in a courteous manner as an individual. You know when someone's attitude towards you is negative and discourteous. It is the same for patients.

The principle of customer service – the ability to supply the customer's wants and needs constantly and consistently – underpins effective patient-centred care. This is important in dentistry as the patient is not always able to assess the standard of clinical work; typically patients can only measure what they can see, feel and hear.

Service is everybody's responsibility in the dental team. To customers, your service attitude is as important as your knowledge and experience. This means managing both the procedures and the customer's experience.

Communication

There are two forms of communication: non–verbal and verbal.

Verbal communication

The following statement has been attributed to several political figures and reflects the issue of what actually makes a good verbal communicator (Fig 3-1):

'I know that you believe you understand what you think I said, but I am not sure you realise that what you heard is not what I meant.'

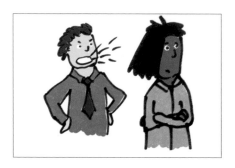

Fig 3-1 Verbal and non-verbal communication.

The key features of good verbal communication include:

- clarity and logic in the way thoughts are presented
- making space for a reply
- using vocabulary and language appropriate for the listener
- good vocal qualities
- asking for feedback on the effectiveness of the message.

Paralinguistic communication – the use of manner of speaking to communicate particular meanings – is a multifactoral aspect of good communication. Paralinguistic communication spans:

- tone : the tone of voice and variation in tone helps to convey information
- volume: different emotions are characterised by changes in volume
- pitch: high pitch is often associated with anger or excitement; low pitch may convey, amongst other attitudes, uncertainty and disinterest
- rate: too fast a speech is often associated with anger; dominance is signalled by slowing down of speech
- 'conversation oil': phrases and vocalisations, for example 'mm-hmm', and 'I see', which fill pauses and gaps in conversations and tend to encourage continuation.

The speed, loudness, tone, timbre and articulation of the spoken voice, coupled with facial expressions and gestures, can be confusing if not misleading to the patient. Inflection can give unintended impressions of aggression, frustration, rudeness or lack of interest. At all times, members of the dental team should strive to communicate in a caring, professional manner that engenders trust and confidence. However, as indicated above, it is not just inflection that leads to effective patient interaction. There are many, varied non-verbal communication methods used across the cultures of the world, with different emphasis and interpretations being placed upon certain postures, signs and gestures. What is entirely acceptable and normal in one culture can be grossly offensive in another. An understanding of these differences is critical to good communication. In the multicultural societies in which most people live and work, it is important to observe, understand and learn about the body language appropriate for different groups. Inappropriate body language can ruin any chance of an effective relationship between a patient and the dental team.

By being aware of non-verbal and verbal communication skills, the dental team can adapt their approaches to ensure that communication with patients is effective, yet remains professional at all times.

Non-verbal communication (Fig 3-2)
As indicated above, there are a number of non-verbal methods of communication (Fig 3-2), some of which may have different meanings in different cultures, for example eye contact between people of different sexes.

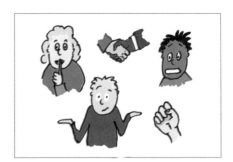

Fig 3-2 Examples of non-verbal communication.

→ *eye contact:* maintaining eye contact helps to build trust in the relationship
→ *body posture:* posture communicates more than words, giving impressions of interest, alertness and purpose
→ *facial expression:* expression can convey emotion; remember if you smile at someone, its difficult for them not to smile back
→ *head movements:* movements of the head can convey that you are acknowledging and listening to what is being said
→ *gesture:* hand movements, ranging from welcoming open hands to clenched fists, can be interpreted in many ways
→ *proximity:* avoid invading people's personal space but standing too far back can come across as standoffish
→ *touch:* tactile people touch other people during communication; this is not always appropriate, let alone welcomed, although it may offer reassurance in some cases.

Equality and diversity

The dental team must be committed to promoting and developing equality and diversity in all its activities. The team must ensure that its ways of working are fair to all individuals and groups, regardless of their origin, race, colour, gender, religion, disability, sexual orientation or age. The modern dental team should have an equality and diversity strategy to help it to tackle discrimination and inequalities. A dental professional must, however, avoid stereotyping patients of different origin, race, colour and so on. Each patient must be treated as an individual, with a strong focus on patient-centred care.

Every patient must be treated as an individual.

Most countries have a multicultural society, increasing in size and expanding in terms of ethnic diversity. As a consequence, dental teams tend to have a diverse mix of patients from many different cultural backgrounds. When providing oral healthcare services to these patients, the responsibility is with the professional to bridge any cultural, ethnic and social divide. It is important that the dental team is aware of, and prepared to manage appropriately, any transcultural issues that may influence the provision of effective care. Under no circumstances should healthcare professionals impose their beliefs and cultural attitudes on a patient.

Language

When members of the dental team and the patient do not share a common language, or when the extent of the common language is limited, there is a substantial risk of failures in patient interaction, some of which may be critical to the management of the patient and clinical outcomes. It is not sufficient to think that the patient understands, or to guess the meaning of patient's responses and questions. In situations in which communication is hampered by lack of a common language, the use of an interpreter, ideally a relative or person accompanying the patient, should be part of the team's management strategy. When using an interpreter, it is important, however, to ensure that patient's confidentiality is not breached and that safeguards are in place to avoid critical issues being lost in translation.

Attitude issues

In seeking to optimise interaction with patients, it is important to recognise that substantial variation exists in attitudes to oral health in modern society. While it is hoped that there is growing appreciation of the importance and benefits of good oral health in all sections of society, it cannot be assumed that every patient shares this appreciation. Assuming that all patients are dentally motivated and aware of the benefits of good oral health runs the risk of poor interaction with those patients most in need of motivation and enlightenment. Such negative effects may be avoided by the dental team being committed to patient-centred care. Where attitudes in respect of oral health are negative, effecting changes in behaviour can be a challenge. To begin to address such challenges, the importance of getting to know and understand the patient through effective interaction cannot be overemphasised. As is often said in respect of diagnosis, listen to the patient for the key to the problem. The same adage applies to attitudes to oral health.

Cultural habits and beliefs

As stressed by Scully and Wilson (2006), an important and expanding aspect of effective patient interaction is knowledge and understanding of cultural habits and beliefs. While acculturisation results in the modification of some habits and beliefs, others are treasured and reinforced, possibly to retain individual and family identity and links to the past. In dealing with such matters, the dental team must always put the interests of the patient first and foremost. As indicated above, under no circumstances should healthcare professionals knowingly or otherwise attempt to impose their cultural habits and belief on a patient, let alone allow their habits and beliefs to compromise the care of the patient.

Positive actions

Developing patient interaction is considered to be an important aspect of a modern approach to oral healthcare provision. Positive actions to achieve this goal include:

- investing time and effort in improving understand of the many facets of the society the dental team serves
- developing practice policies to ensure that all patients, and members of the dental team, will be treated fairly, equally and with respect
- seeking feedback from patients, including suggestions for ways to improve interactions in the future; constructive criticism can be a very valuable resource
- keeping meticulous, contemporary records of any incidents, particularly any that caused a breakdown in team–patient relationships; learn from mistakes and complaints
- observing how other organisations deal with the dental team
- adopting good practice and seeking to develop a culture of continuous quality improvement
- developing practice leaflets, websites and other materials to meet the needs of the clientele.

Trust and confidence

Patients should have trust and confidence in their dental healthcare professionals. The dental team–patient relationship, which is one of the pillars of trust and confidence in caring for patients, must be a professional one, as must be relationships within the dental team. Such relationships must never be abused, let alone taken for granted, as this will destroy trust and confidence. In the absence trust and confidence, dental care will, at best, be compromised. Gone are the days when patients have unquestioning trust and confidence in healthcare professionals. Patients increasingly expect those caring for them to demonstrate their professionalism and capacity to deal with their problems in a fit and proper manner. Effective patient interaction is central to satisfying these expectations.

> Patient's trust and confidence is earned, possibly even hard won, and must be valued and preserved.

Reference

Scully C, Wilson NHF. Culturally Sensitive Oral Healthcare. [Quintessentials of Dental Practice series, Vol. 35.] London: Quintessence, 2006.

Further reading and useful websites

British Dental Association: www.bda.org.

General Dental Council: www.gdc-uk.org.

Medical Protection Society: www.mps.org.uk.

Chapter 4
Handling patient complaints: negative to positive outcomes

Gail Vernon

Aim

This chapter aims to emphasise the rights of patients to complain and the ways in which complaints should be managed and viewed as positives rather than negatives.

Outcome

In addition to considering the steps to be taken in responding to complaints, this chapter is intended to give the dental team a positive approach to the successful management of concerns, criticisms and complaints.

Introduction: recognising imperfection

In addition to it being unrealistic to expect to please all patients all of the time, it is important for members of the dental team to recognise, individually and collectively, that no one is perfect. As a consequence, everyone will, from time to time, be the subject of a complaint, or at least some level of criticism, irrespective of how hard individuals and the team try to behave and perform in an ideal manner. Complaints and criticisms should not therefore be treated defensively, but as events, unwelcome as they may be, as a stimulus to review, audit and, where appropriate, take action to modify behaviours, procedures and techniques. Whilst recognising that the occasional complaint can be vexatious, caution must be exercised in dismissing any complaint, irrespective how trivial. Not to accept some criticism, possibly in the form of a complaint, could be considered foolhardy.

Complaints can be opportunities

It might not be immediately understood, but complaints should be looked upon as an opportunity to correct, or possibly just improve matters, with positive outcomes. It is important to capitalise on these opportunities, enhance the services provided to patients and, as a consequence, reduce the risk of similar complaints in the future.

If a patient is unhappy with the service or treatment they receive, it is to be hoped that they make their feelings known, and the dental team has the opportunity to address the situation. The alternative is that patient severs their link with the practice, and may make it their business to tell friends and family, if not various agencies, about their loss of trust and confidence in the service provided by the dental team. Under such circumstances, resolving matters can become exceedingly difficult, if not impossible, and the dental team tends to be faced with damage limitation rather than the prospect of any positive outcomes.

Professional responsibility requires you to answer complaints satisfactorily, put matters right, and use the information provided to improve your service. With this in mind, the dental team should have a complaints procedure in place that the team is familiar with and trained to deliver, as and when the need arises. As recommended by various professional organisations, nationally and internationally, the initial management of any complaint should involve listening to the complainant, recording the complaint, acknowledging any failings and limitations which have occurred and seeking ways to resolve the issue locally at the practice level, thereby avoiding the need for a formal, typically stressful investigation by a third party. Very often resolution can be achieved by making an apology and agreeing arrangements to put things right. Some complaints can, however, be difficult to resolve. Such difficulties tend to arise when the patient has experienced pain, distress or inconvenience for which they expect compensation, or believe reflects negligence, if not incompetence in the way they have been treated. Complaints of such a serious nature are best dealt with by third parties. One of the skills in the successful management of complaints is knowing when to seek help and support, albeit that it escalates the matter to involve external agencies.

What do patients expect when making a complaint?

When making a complaint, a patient usually wants to know a number of things.

* What has happened?
* Why it happened?
* What will be done to put it right?
* Whether anyone is to blame?
* What action will be taken to ensure it doesn't happen again?

In answering these questions, honesty and transparency can greatly assist the opportunity for local resolution. Even if a patient is angry or distressed there is usually at least some acceptance of an oversight or inadvertent error. When patients sense that their complaint is not being dealt with openly and truthfully, then they can become increasingly unwilling to consider local resolution.

The complaint procedure

A complaint from a patient should trigger a well-rehearsed procedure by members of the dental team (Fig 4-1).

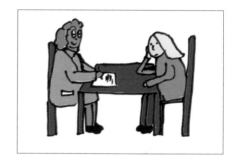

Fig 4-1 The importance of listening, recording and sympathy in the complaints procedure.

There is great merit in the team having identified a senior member of the team to deal with all complaints. This individual, ideally someone training in the management of complaints, should be familiar with all aspects of the activities of the team.

With the complainant taken aside, preferably to an office or other enclosed room, and reassured that their complaint will be dealt with promptly and thoroughly, the person dealing with the complaint should do the following: listen, sympathise, do not justify and agree on a course of action. It is then essential to follow-through on the complaint and to ensure that the person making the complaint understands that this will happen and that they will be kept informed.

Listen

It is important to listen in a way that reassures a complainant that what they are saying is being taken in and considered. The use of body language and physical prompts to show listening are also important. In addition, it is helpful to the complainant to see notes being made of the details of the complaint. If, however, the complaint is in respect of personal matters, it is important to seek the approval of the complainant to make notes. In such circumstances, confidentiality must be respected. It costs nothing to listen, and the more attentive the listener is, the more it will diffuse the situation. Furthermore, by listening carefully, it often becomes clear what actions the complainant considers necessary to resolve the situation.

Sympathise
Sympathising is not the same as agreeing; it does not mean accepting liability or a signal that you are open to all sorts of criticism. What it does is take the heat out of the situation. A few well-chosen words reaffirm that the complainant is being listened to and there is no attempt to belittle or duck the situation. For example, saying 'I'm really sorry to hear what you are telling me; please tell me more so that I can fully understand the problem' should help to temper what the patient goes on to complain about.

Do not justify
The irate person is often not the least bit interested in excuses such as the dental team being short staffed through illness. Such things are not their problem. Whatever possible reasons the dental team may have for things having gone wrong, they are not a justification. As and when it comes to putting matters right, there may be opportunity to explain the reasons for the difficulties to the complainant. Complainants are much more likely to be understanding of unforeseen circumstances and events when they have received an apology and steps are being taken to put things right.

Make records
If complainants see that records are being made of their complaint, together with agreed actions and suggestions as to how arrangements could be improved, they tend to be reassured. Furthermore, as and when it comes to writing to a complainant to give an update on actions taken or, hopefully, draw a line under the complaint, records are invaluable in ensuring that factual inaccuracies do not creep in, giving the patient further good cause to complain.

Agree on a course of action
Having listened, sympathised and made notes, what next? Normally, subject to the complaint having been well managed and the complainant reassured, it is appropriate to proceed to ask one of the following questions.

- How do you think we should take this forward?
- How would you like me to handle this from here?
- How do you see us resolving this situation?

The answers to such questions should point to the way out of the situation. While it may not be the wish of the team to capitulate to all the demands of the complainant, it is often a small price to pay to meet all the reasonable expectations, and thereby have opportunity to achieve closure on the complaint. Meeting the expectations of a complaint does not mean accepting liability, or opting for the easy, albeit possibly costly, way out of the situation. Needless to say, unrealistic expectations should be identified as matters needing further discussion. Confrontation should always be avoided in such circumstances.

Follow through
Follow through is pivotal to the successful outcome of managing a complaint. Without follow through, the actions already taken may be to no avail. Telephone calls must be returned, commitments must be kept, letters sent according to agreed actions, arrangements changed in the practice and so on, otherwise complainants tend to feel that they have been misled, adding insult to injury. In this regard, agreed actions should not include commitments that cannot be honoured.

Risk management

An integral element of managing complaints is to learn from mistakes and to adopt a risk management approach to making the dental team less likely to be the subject of future complaints.

There are various steps dental professionals can take to reduce the risk of complaints, including the following.

- Keep patients informed about issues, in particular delays to treatment, changes to treatment plans and the anticipated outcome of the treatment.
- Avoid technical terms and jargon when talking to patients. If patients fail to understand their treatment and what it will achieve, the risk of complaints is greatly increased. In such considerations, it is important to remember that patients, in particular those with limited language skills, are reluctant to admit that they do not understand what they have been told.

- Be clear with patients about contractual arrangements. Inform patients of the basis and charge of a consultation when offering an appointment.
- Provide a detailed written plan and fee estimate to avoid confusion, in particular for complex, expensive treatments.
- Obtain informed consent and include it in the patient's records prior to commencing treatment.
- Provide pre- and post-treatment patient information leaflets, explaining what will happen, what to expect and what to do in the event of concerns and unexpected complications.
- Ensure arrangements are in place for emergency cover, including clear instructions to patients as to who to contact for emergency care.
- Avoid making unrealistic or ambiguous claims or commitments.

Given that well-founded complaints are improvements waiting to happen, patients who make genuine complaints should be viewed as an asset rather than a threat and, as such, should be well looked after rather than being treated as a nuisance, or with suspicion and disdain.

Effective handling of patient complaints can be a real 'practice-builder': turning negatives into positives.

> Well-founded complaints are improvements waiting to happen.

Further reading and useful websites

Dental Defence Union: www.the–ddu.com

General Dental Council: www.gdc-uk.org

Lilley R. Dealing with Difficult People. London: Kogan Page, 2002.

Chapter 5

Making the working environment safe

Nairn Wilson

Aim

The aim of this chapter is to familiarise the dental team with an outline of the measures to make the working environment safe. This includes general issues, personal protection and instrument safety.

Outcome

The chapter should lead to an understanding of the importance of a safe working environment and how it may be best achieved, including methods to protect the members of the dental team and methods to ensure that instruments are clean and sterile.

Safety in general

Nairn Wilson

There are many aspects to safety in the working environment. These include processes and requirements common to any working environment, such as fire precautions, electrical safety and the safe use of equipment, together with many other measures devised to protect both those who work in the environment and others who visit the workplace for whatever purpose. There are, in addition, processes and requirements for specific types of workplace, with clinical workplace environments being no exception. In the clinical workplace, and in particular environments for the provision of oral healthcare, there are many varied processes and requirements, which vary in their nature and extent according to the type of patient being treated and the treatment provided. These processes and requirements may vary nationally and internationally, but they are increasingly the subject of international guidance and common expectations of good practice.

In this chapter, special attention is paid to two areas, personal protection and the decontamination of instruments in the dental clinical environment, with an emphasis on the dental practice rather than the hospital or other community-based clinical environment. This emphasis is not intended to belittle or otherwise down-play the critical importance of other aspects of safety in the dental workplace environment. The other aspects of safety in the dental workplace include safety in respect of the use of ionising radiation and pressure vessels; the storage and dispensing of drugs; the dispatch and receipt of clinical materials, including work to be sent and received from the dental laboratory; the storage, use and disposal of hazardous substances; and special safety precautions for patients with special needs. The reader is referred to relevant legislation, national and international guidance and other literature that deal with such matters in detail. Keeping abreast of all relevant developments in respect of safety is challenging.

As a guiding principle, the working environment should pose no threat to anyone who works in it or has occasion to visit it. Workers and visitors should feel safe and secure in the workplace environment, free of any feelings of unrecognised, uncontrolled dangers and hazards. Safety in the workplace should be the subject of regular audit and risk assessment, possibly involving external assessments and other form of inspection. Safety is difficult to ensure in a clinical environment that is outdated or poorly maintained. Modern design and facilities greatly assist the management of safety issues.

Irrespective of care and attention paid to safety, there is always some risk of untoward events. To be prepared to deal with such events, there should be provisions and training in the workplace for matters ranging from first aid, including basic life support, to procedures to be followed in the event of a major incident such as a fire.

Safety in the workplace is an individual and collective responsibility. All relevant safety procedures and arrangements should be second nature to the dental team. To achieve this, the dental team should develop detailed written protocols that are both kept up to date and rehearsed from time to time, ideally on a regular basis.

Safety is not an option, it is fundamental to modern clinical practice and to fulfilling one of the dental team's principal professional responsibilities: protection of the patient.

> Safety in the workplace should be the subject of regular audit and risk assessment.

Safety in the workplace is an individual and collective responsibility.

Safety is not an option, it is fundamental to modern clinical practice.

Personal protection

Gail Vernon

Introduction

With the emergence of new infectious diseases and increasing prevalence of blood-borne viral diseases, including HIV and hepatitis B and C, the importance of personal protection in the dental clinical environment has grown dramatically. Depending on local and national requirements, all clinical members of the dental team may need to be successfully immunised against diphtheria, hepatitis B, pertussis, poliomyelitis, rubella, tetanus and tuberculosis.

'Super bugs', microorganisms resistant to many of the usual antimicrobial agents, and their impact on healthcare continue to have a high media profile. As a result, patients are increasing aware of infection risks in clinical environments and the requirements of health professionals to observe infection control procedures. This increased awareness leaves patients expecting to observe such activities when visiting healthcare environments; dental surgeries are no exception.

A key element of infection control recommended by authorities worldwide is the concept of standard precautions as a means to reduce disease transmission. The primary concept is that all patients are potentially infectious, as most carriers of infection are unaware of their condition.

This necessitates the implementation of a comprehensive infection control procedure. The World Dental Federation recommends that all oral health professionals adhere to standard precautions as set by the local or regional authorities, as appropriate.

Every dental practice, hospital and laboratory will have a written infection control policy tailored to their individual routines.

Employers have a duty to ensure that all members of staff are satisfactorily trained. This training should include:

- how infections are transmitted
- preparing a practice policy on decontamination and infection control
- what personal protection is required and when to use it
- what to do in the event of accidents or personal injury.

The entire dental team is responsible for implementing, complying and keeping up to date in respect of infection control procedures.

The information relating to infection control procedures is wide ranging. This section provides an introduction to policies that may impact on the personnel of the dental team. This information is, however, by no means exhaustive and further reading is recommended.

History taking and confidentiality
Dental professionals have an ethical obligation to provide treatment for all patients. As a consequence, infection control policies must be universally applied; this is of particular importance given that most carriers of latent disease are unaware of their condition and some patients may not wish to disclose information at all. Patient information and the medical history help in assessing any risks of potential infection to the dental team and other patients.

From this information, procedures in line with standard precautions can be implemented to protect practice staff, patients and laboratory personnel. Any disclosures by the patients must be treated confidentially and should not be passed to any other party without the prior consent of the patient. The matter of disclosure and confidentiality is further expanded in Chapter 3.

A medical history must always be taken at the first visit to the practice and should be updated on a regular basis. All relevant information must be carefully recorded as part of the patient's clinical record and updated as appropriate.

Personal and team protection
All members of the dental team need to understand the principles of personal protection and comply with relevant policies, including those pertaining to immunisation. Personal protection involves a range of measures.

Protective clothing
Protective clothing includes uniforms, which will have certain material requirements for safety, and various items for specific purposes. At times, protective clothing is a personal choice; however, the following points should be considered.

The material forming the protective clothing should be capable of withstanding temperatures of 65°C to allow for effective washing to eliminate any potential microbial contamination. The style of the protective clothing may vary according to the procedures being undertaken and the potential for contamination. Increasingly, chairside personnel are adopting short-sleeved tunics or tops, leaving the forearms bare. This facilitates washing of the hands, including the wrists and forearms, and is most acceptable to patients. When undertaking procedures that involve the production of large amounts of splatter or aerosol contaminated with saliva or blood, the protective clothing may be protected by a disposable, single-use plastic apron, which covers the thighs in the sitting position. Given such measures, a protective tunic or top may itself be worn for a whole clinical session, possibly even a day, unless it becomes frankly contaminated or otherwise soiled.

Protective clothing should not be worn outside the practice or hospital environment. Long-sleeved gowns, increasingly of a disposable, single-use type, continue to be used for surgical procedures. Such gowns are donned after scrubbing-up and prior to putting on single-use, disposable, sterile surgical gloves.

Other protective clothing should include footwear that will protects the feet from falling instruments and made of a material that is non-absorbent, ideally with a smooth, shiny, impervious surface. It is good practice to change out of outdoor footwear into clinical footwear prior to a clinical session.

Eye protection
Safety glasses should be worn by all members of the dental team and patients (Fig 5-1). Safety glasses help to protect eyes against trauma and contamination from foreign bodies, splatter and droplets in aerosols. Prescription glasses, if worn by the patient, should be removed and replaced by protective glasses. If the chairside members of the dental team wear prescription glasses, the options are the use of a facial shield (visor), which many clinicians prefer to the use of protective glasses, the use of protective glasses that cover the prescription glasses, or the use of protective glasses including prescription lenses. Whatever form of eye or facial protection is used, it is important to

47

have side protection, provided by side wings to the protective glasses or a facial shield curving round the side of the face. If the operator wishes to use loupes, these should be fixed to the protective eyewear. Facial shields should be changed between patients. The surfaces of protective glasses need to be thoroughly cleaned with a surface disinfectant between patients, care being taken to avoid residual disinfectant on the glasses, which could irritate the eye. Protective eyewear should be worn as a matter or routine while undertaking laboratory work

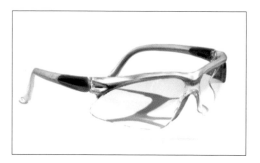

Fig 5-1 Safety glasses. (Reproduced from Martin et al. 2009.)

Face protection
A close-fitting face mask that covers the nose and mouth should be worn by all chairside members of the dental team when undertaking all forms of treatment. Face masks must be changed between patients and as and when they become moist during a prolonged procedure. Members of the dental team working in the dental laboratory should wear a face mask whenever generating dust and aerosols.

Hand protection
Good hand hygiene is the single most important infection control measure. Chairside members of the dental team should wash their hands with a detergent or liquid soap intended for clinical use:

* whenever the hands become soiled, dirty or contaminated
* before and after eating and drinking
* before and after going to the toilet
* after coughing, sneezing or nose blowing
* after touching, rubbing or scratching skin or hair
* when starting or completing clinical sessions.

The technique for routine hand washing is illustrated in Fig 5-2. It is important to remove all jewellery, wrist watches and other items prior to all clinical sessions, the only possible exception being a simple, smooth-surfaced, narrow wedding band. If a nailbrush is used, it should be single-use.

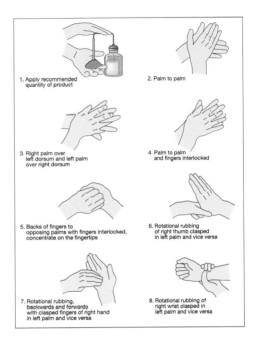

Fig 5-2 The Ayliffe technique for systematic handwashing. (Reproduced from Martin et al. 2009.)

Between patients, or at other times when changing gloves, the hands can be decontaminated with an appropriate, typically alcohol-containing, hand rub or gel, assuming that the hands have not suffered frank contamination, for which hand washing is indicated.

Gloves should be worn when in contact with the patient, handling items that are contaminated, when preparing and cleaning down clinical areas, when handling clinical waste and when dealing with any clinical spillages. Gloves should be treated as single-use and discarded when leaving the operating area or wishing to handle items such as the patient's clinical record, radiographs and related items, including writing implements. Used gloves should be regarded as clinical waste. Given the increasing incidence and potential life-threatening nature of allergic reactions to latex, it is good practice to use non-latex single-use disposable gloves.

Cracked, lacerated or abraded skin increases the risk of microorganisms entering through the skin. Any cuts or abrasions should be covered with waterproof plasters. Regular use of an emollient hand cream prevents the hands from drying. Ideally, good-quality moisturising hand cream should be used after the end of each session.

Sharps injuries

Sharps injuries are a likely route for transmission of blood-borne viral infections in dentistry. Sharps injuries are caused through inadvertent penetration of the skin with a contaminated object in the form of a needle, instrument or dental appliance.

Despite the introduction of different forms of syringes to eliminate, or at least reduce, the risk of sharps injuries, such injuries, despite care, do occasionally happen. In the event of a sharps injury, the first aid includes:

- encourage bleeding from the wound, typically a puncture site
- wash the area thoroughly with soap and water under running water; the wound should not be scrubbed
- dry the wound with disposable paper towels
- cover the wound with a waterproof dressing.

Following successful completion of first aid, it is good practice to have the patient agree to a blood test to ascertain if the patient has any risk factors for blood-borne viruses. Such tests are voluntary, but greatly assist in dealing with the sharps injury.

To limit the risk of sharp injuries, all members of the dental team must be trained in the safe disposal of sharps in a sharps bins (Fig 5-3).

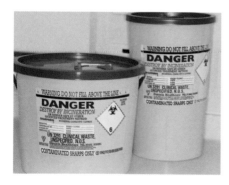

Fig 5-3 Sharps bins. Courtesy of Dr Chris Dickinson.

Environment

The surgery layout and design plays a vital part in infection control. The chair, work and floor surfaces should be made from an impervious material. All equipment included in the surgery should be fit for the purpose and be able to be adequately protected, decontaminated or sterilised prior to use, between patients or before repair.

Zoning within the surgery will allow clear identification of areas of high, medium and low risk, and areas for decontamination, sterilisation and specific procedures such as imaging assuming such activities are carried out in the surgery.

Zoning areas in the surgery simplifies the decontamination process. The risk areas are those that may be contaminated during use and should be cleaned and disinfected between patients. Barrier coverings should be used to cover such items as light handles, the chair headrest, handpiece tubing and control panels, which cannot be adequately decontaminated. These coverings must be changed between patients, with the surfaces being cleaned between the removal of decontaminated coverings and the placement of fresh coverings. Barrier coverings limit the contamination of surfaces in a manner similar to the way in which gloves prevent contamination of the hands. Barrier coverings greatly reduce, but may not eliminate contamination of surfaces. Any surfaces found or suspected to be contaminated must be decontaminated.

Disposal of contaminated waste

All waste in the dental practice or laboratory, other than sharps, which must be disposed of in sharps bins, should be separated into clinical and non-clinical waste. Clinical waste contains contaminated items that may prove hazardous to any other person, including, gloves, cotton wool rolls, swabs, bibs and any other items contaminated with saliva, blood or other body fluids. Clinical waste, all of which should be classified as hazardous waste, must be stored securely in appropriate bags or other containers, such as sharps bins, according to local requirements and collected by a registered waste carrier, typically for high temperature incineration. Waste radiographic fixer and developer solutions are hazardous and should be safely stored awaiting collection by a suitably licensed company.

Regarding waste disposal, as with all aspects of safety in the working environment, all members of the dental team should make themselves aware of all relevant laws and regulations. If ever in doubt, advice should be sought.

Decontamination of dental instruments

Michael Martin

Introduction

Dental instruments can become heavily contaminated with blood and saliva and be a potential source of infection to members of the dental team and patients. It is, therefore, very important that they are properly decontaminated and that the process is done safely. A large number of sharps injuries occur when instrument are cleaned. This process needs careful thought, planning and practice if these injuries are not to occur. Since the cleaning process has the potential for sharps injuries and blood–to–blood contact, it is vital that personnel involved in decontamination have been effectively vaccinated, in particular against hepatitis B.

Decontamination

Decontamination is a term that is often misused, as it does not just mean the removal of contaminants. It is defined as the removal or destruction of microbial contaminants to render the instrument safe for reuse. Thus the term decontamination includes cleaning and sterilisation. In addition, the term decontamination increasingly tends to encompass the safe storage of instruments. Unless an instrument is completely clean, it cannot be sterilised, or be considered safe for use. If blood, or other material, is left on an instrument prior to sterilisation, microorganisms present could be protected and remain viable. In addition, proteins or other detritus left on instruments can cause damage in surgical wounds, as they act as foreign matter. It is, therefore, vitally important that invasive surgical instruments are properly cleaned and sterilised prior to reuse.

> Unless an instrument is completely clean, it cannot be sterilised or be considered safe for use.

Assessment of instruments for risk

Some pieces of equipment become heavily contaminated with saliva and blood and always need decontamination; these are called critical instruments. Other equipment, for example protective glasses, bib chains and face mirrors, should not be mixed up with critical instruments and do not need decontamination, just cleaning as they are not used for invasive procedures. The careful separation of critical instruments, which are used for invasive procedures, is the first step in organising decontamination procedures. This can save both time and effort. Another part of the planning of decontamination is the consideration of the use of disposable instruments. Many pieces of equipment, for example inserts for high-vacuum saliva ejectors, are very difficult to clean and, as such, are best bought as single-use disposable items. The judicious use of disposable items may at first seem costly, but it often can save staff time and, in turn costs. Other pieces of equipment, for example endodontic files, are designed to be used only once and are marked by the manufacturers with a symbol to signify single use (Fig 5-4). Such items must not be reused as they are often incapable of being effectively decontaminated.

Before any critical reusable item is purchased, it is essential to have the manufacturer state how it should be decontaminated. Many manufacturers do not specify this information or refer the purchaser, often vaguely, to the current generic guidelines; it is best not to buy such instruments.

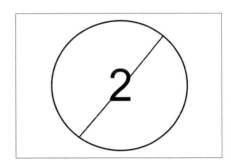

Fig 5-4 The international symbol indicating single-use instruments. (Reproduced from Martin et al. 2009.)

Instrument cleaning
Instruments can be cleaned in four ways, manually, with enzymes, ultrasonically and with washer/disinfectors. The merits of each of these will be considered.

Manual cleaning
Manual cleaning is by far the most widely used method for cleaning dental instruments. It is also the least-efficient cleaning method and the most dangerous. All dental instruments that have been used for invasive procedures are dangerous after use; they have blood on them and they are sharp. Manual cleaning, therefore, involves some risk of a sharps injury and is, as a consequence, strongly discouraged. Studies on the amount of residual

debris left after systematic manual washing show that cleaning of instruments is operator and time variable; it has no place in safe dental practice.

> All dental instruments that have been used for invasive procedures are dangerous after use.

Enzyme cleaning
There are a whole variety of enzyme cleaners available for dental use. None of those currently available removes prions, the causative agents of Creutzfeldt–Jakob disease. Enzyme cleaners can be useful either as an initial cleaning agent or as a place for 'holding' soiled instruments, in particular those heavily contaminated with blood. 'Holding' tanks are especially useful to prevent blood and other material from drying on instruments. Blood and saliva is very much more difficult to remove once it has dried. Enzyme cleaners are best supplemented with another method such as ultrasonics or washer disinfectors to ensure complete cleaning.

Ultrasonic cleaning
Ultrasonic cleaners are extensively used in dental practice, and also extensively abused. Ultrasonics works by creating 'planes' of water in the tank that have vacuums between them. When these planes collapse, they release energy that dislodges material from the surface of the instrument. There are several very important practical points in the use of ultrasonics.

- Before use, the tank should be set up properly and tested by an expert to ensure it works. This is called commissioning; it is essential.
- The manufacturer's recommended cleaning time for the instruments in the tank must be adhered to without interruption. Unless this is followed precisely, then instruments will not be cleaned. Instruments should never be added to a part-cleaned load.
- The tank should not be overloaded and liquid must flow freely around all the instruments. The clear flow of liquid around instruments ensures that they are cleaned on all surfaces.
- All instruments must be visually inspected at the end of the cycle to ensure that they are clean.
- The tank must be emptied regularly, at least after every session and if heavily used more frequently.

- The fluid used in the tank must be that recommended by the manufacturer; ideally one containing a detergent. Disinfectants, unless combined with a detergent and recommended by the manufacturer, should not be used in ultrasonic baths: disinfectants change proteins and help them to stick on to instruments.
- The liquids used in ultrasonic tanks need careful degassing before use. This is simply done by running the ultrasonic bath with cleaning liquid in it, according to manufacturer's directions, prior to use.
- Records should be kept of all ultrasonic use. Units fitted with a printer are to be preferred.
- Staff should be trained and audited in ultrasonic cleaning.

Ultrasonic baths are precision instruments that need careful monitoring to ensure appropriate working, and testing for their cleaning efficiency.

The simplest test to ensure that an ultrasonic bath is working is the foil ablation test. Strips of kitchen foil, weighted down with paper clips to ensure that they hang vertically, are placed in the bath water in as many places as possible (Fig 5-5a). The bath is run for its normal cycle without interruption and the strips are then examined (Fig 5-5b). If the bath is working correctly, the strips should show extensive wear and destruction. If the strips are not damaged, the bath should not be used and sent for repair. The most likely cause of failure is that the ultrasonic transducer has become disconnected from the bath. Ultrasonic cleaners can also be tested with special probes that which measure the ultrasonic waves in the bath, but these are expensive and need expert use. The foil ablation test should be done at least weekly if the tank is heavily used.

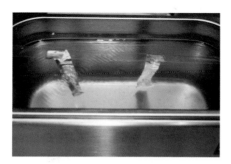 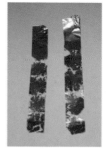

Fig 5-5 Foil ablation test. (a) Strips of kitchen foil, weighted down with paper clips to ensure they hang vertically, are placed in the bath water in as many places as possible. (b) The strips are examined after the bath has run for its normal cycle without interruption. (Reproduced from Martin et al. 2009.)

At least every month the efficiency of the cleaning power of the tank should be tested. The best way of testing this is to contaminate an instrument with a test 'soil'. This is usually a mixture of blood and albumin. The test soil is painted on an instrument, which is then placed in the bath and the cycle activated to completion without interruption. After the cycle is completed, the amount of soil left on the instrument is estimated with a ninhydrin test. Ninhydrin is a reagent that changes colour in the presence of protein. The amount of colour indicates how much protein is present. Practically, these tests are done by wiping a moist swab over the instrument to remove any residual soil and then plunging it into ninhydrin (Fig 5-6). If protein is present, the swab will be discoloured. The instrument should be clean and have no residual protein present at the end of the cycle. If the ultrasonic bath fails this test, it should not be used and sent for repair. Tests of this kind are called validation tests, as they assess whether the machine works; results should always be recorded.

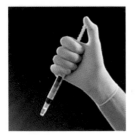 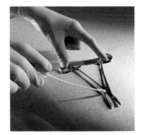 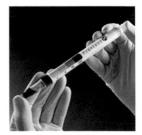

Fig 5-6 The ninhydrin test. (a) A simple residual protein-testing kit includes swab and reagent. (b) The swab is rubbed over the surface of a washed instrument to collect any residual protein. (c) The swab is submerged in reagent and colour is allowed to develop. The intensity of colour change is proportional to the amount of protein present. (Reproduced from Martin et al. 2009, courtesy of Medisafe Ltd.)

Washer disinfectors
Washer disinfectors are machines designed to clean dental instruments reproducibly. The machines first flush the instruments in cold water, with agitation from high-power jets to remove most of the adherent debris; hot water would coagulate any blood present. The instruments are then washed in detergent and hot water before being thoroughly rinsed several times. Some machines then heat the instruments to 80°C for 10 minutes or 90°C for 1 minute: this is called thermal disinfection as it kills many residual microorganisms. Finally, the instruments are dried. Once the process is

complete, the instruments should be inspected and if necessary rewashed if not visibly clean. Washer disinfectors do take time to complete their cycles: commonly at least 40 minutes. While instruments are being cleaned, they are out of action and so these machines create a need for significantly more instruments in the practice. Washer disinfectors also require a clean supply of water. This water can be supplied by a reverse osmosis machine or by passing mains water through an ion-exchange resin.

Washer disinfectors have to be commissioned to ensure that they work properly. In addition, they need to be routinely tested. At the start of each day, the machine should be run without any instruments in it and the manufacturer's parameters checked on the printout (wash cycle times, temperature of wash, thermal disinfection times etc.); this is called a process check. The rotor arms in the machine should be checked for blockages and free movement and the internal drum cleaned. Once a week, a validation test should be done with an instrument contaminated with a test soil and the amount of residual protein estimated with the ninhydrin test as described above.

> Washer disinfectors are the preferred means for cleaning dental instruments.

Sterilisation

Sterilisation is the killing of all forms of life including prions. In dentistry, this is achieved by using superheated steam. Increasing the pressure of steam allows it to hold more heat; this is called latent heat. The instrument that is used for sterilising instruments is the autoclave. Steam is generated in the autoclave and pumped into a central chamber. If the steam is used to displace the air in the chamber, it is called a type N autoclave and should be used for solid instruments only. Type N autoclaves have steam and residual air in their chambers and, consequently, the heat generated cannot penetrate small tubes. So these autoclaves are limited in use to solid instruments. If air is displaced from the central chamber by pumping it out and steam is then pumped in, the superheated steam can penetrate items such as handpieces. Autoclaves utilising this process are called type S, or specific load autoclaves. Autoclaves which pump most of the air out and have a high saturation of steam can sterilise instruments with a small lumen; these are called type B autoclaves. In dentistry, the ideal autoclave is a type B autoclave, but most instruments can be sterilised by use of a type S machine. Once the autoclave is in use, it is important that the necessary pressure is maintained for the required time if sterilisation is to be achieved. The recommended combinations of time, temperature and pressure are:

- 134°C for 3 minutes at 2 bar
- 115°C for 30 minutes at 1 bar
- 121°C for 15 minutes at 1 bar.

Autoclaves need to be filled with clean water and the reservoirs regularly cleaned. Ideally, water in autoclaves should be used once only, but older types reuse the water. These latter types need frequent cleaning.

Autoclaves must be commissioned before use and checked and validated. Each day, they should be run empty before use to ensure that the correct temperature time and pressure combinations are achieved. The most accurate method of validating proper function is with an indwelling thermocouple. Most autoclaves have this facility. In some countries, biological indicators are used to check autoclaves. These indicators, filled with heat-resistant spores of *Geobacillus stearothermophillus*, are put into the autoclave. The biological indicator is incubated at room temperature after sterilisation for three to four days. If there is no growth, then sterilisation has been achieved.

Autoclaves need careful loading to ensure the free circulation of steam around the instruments. The chamber and door seals need regular cleaning as they can get soiled, in particular with oil from handpieces.

Storage of instruments
All decontaminated instruments should be stored aseptically in containers, wrapped in paper, pouches or sterilisation bags. Instruments should be stored dry. All forms of life, including microorganisms, require water for life, hence lack of it prevents them growing. In addition, wet instruments can corrode. Hinged instruments must be stored open to prevent corrosion in and around the hinge. Storing hinged instruments, such as pliers, open also prevents electrolytic corrosion between the beaks. A variety of autoclavable tray systems can be used for instrument kits. Such systems are ideal for instrument storage. Pouches and sterilisation bags are best used for instruments that are used intermittently, such as elevators and luxators. Pouches and bags are only suitable for type B and some type S autoclaves. Instruments should never be stored loose in drawers or cupboards, as they will become contaminated.

Dental handpieces

Dental handpieces are very difficult to clean because they have a number of tubes with small lumens, together with an intricate bearing. Traditionally, dental handpieces were cleaned by squirting oil into them from aerosol cans; this approach to cleaning is now considered to be ineffective. The only satisfactory method of cleaning handpieces is to use a mechanical device, together with alcohols to clean the bearings and detergents to clean the water jets. These machines are expensive, but they more than save their cost in lengthening the life of the handpiece bearing. If handpieces are not cleaned properly, adherent material gets baked onto the handpiece bearing during sterilisation. This causes the bearing to spin eccentrically and, as a consequence, to wear. Cleaning the bearing properly avoids this problem and prolongs the bearing's life. Clean handpieces need a type S or B autoclave to sterilise them, as the steam in these machines can penetrate the fine lumens within the handpieces.

Creation of a central or in-surgery local decontamination area

If there are a number of operators working in a practice, and there is space, then a central decontamination area could be considered. Central decontamination areas have advantages, including:

- decontamination equipment can be shared
- all the noise and steam is generated away from the surgery
- processes can be validated in one area
- more space is available in the surgery.

But there are disadvantages:

- the capital cost of the equipment may be high
- dedicated staff are required to work in central decontamination areas
- members of the dental team tend not to enjoy prolonged periods of working in these areas
- many more instruments are required
- instruments have to be transported safely to and from the central decontamination area.

If local in-surgery decontamination is used, then it must be designed carefully and contain the following areas:

- a 'dirty' receiving area
- a cleaning area, containing a washer/disinfector or ultrasonic machine and a handpiece cleaner

- an inspection area with a light/magnifier, together with a sink for cleaning instruments that are still soiled; this sink should not be used for handwashing or other purposes
- a sterilisation area containing autoclaves
- a storage area.

There should be no 'clutter' in local decontamination areas, which require a clear direction of throughput of instruments from dirty to clean. Benching should be covered, if adjacent to a wall, and amenable to effective cleaning.

Conclusions

Safety in the workplace should be the subject of regular audit and risk assessment and seen as both an individual and a collective responsibility.

Personal safety involves awareness of general potential hazards and specific hazards; the latter may be identified from taking a good history but it cannot be assumed that all will be known about every patient.

The dental team and patients need protective clothing that is suitable for the particular task, including specific aprons, bibs, glasses and gloves. Members of the dental team need to have good hand washing techniques and to be aware of the potential danger of injury from sharps.

Decontamination is the preparation of invasive instruments for reuse and involves cleaning and sterilisation. Unless an instrument is clean it cannot be sterilised.

There are a number of machines that are used for decontaminating and sterilising instruments and these must be properly commissioned and validated.

Decontamination areas must be carefully designed to ensure clear separation of clean and dirty areas.

Further reading and useful websites

British Dental Association: www.bda-dentistry.org.uk

General Dental Council: www.gdc-uk.org,

Health & Safety Executive: www.hse.gov.uk

Martin MV, Fulford MR, Preston AJ. Infection Control for the Dental Team. Quintessentials of General Dental Practice, vol 39.] London: Quintessence, 2009.

Walker JT, Dickenson J, Sutton JM, Raven ND, Marsh PD. Cleanability of dental instruments: implications of residual protein and risks of Creutzfeldt–Jakob disease. Br Dent J 2007;203:395-401.

World Dental Federation: www.fdiworldental.org/

Chapter 6
Culture of the workplace
The workplace

Carole Brennan and Marina Harris

Aim

The aim of this chapter is to understand the different types of organisational culture in the workplace and their effects on the individuals working within them.

Outcome

After reading this chapter, readers should have an awareness of different organisational cultures that can exist in the dental workplace and be able to appreciate that matching the organisational culture with a preferred team role and personality can enhance an individual's enjoyment of their work and assist in achieving professional goals.

Introduction

Most members of the dental team have worked in more than one dental practice, clinic laboratory, department, university or company. Indeed, most members of the dental team have worked in various settings in their professional lives.

When a person moves to a different place of work, having changed jobs, transferred to a different laboratory or department or acquired a different practice, it is typical to be struck by the different atmosphere: the ways of doing things, the different pace of working, the relationships between members of the dental team, the individual responsibilities and the different personalities. This is possibly not surprising given that organisations are as different and varied as the nations and societies of the world. They have different cultures: sets of values, norms and beliefs reflected in different structures and systems and influenced by many different variables.

On reflection, most people will, in all probability, have experienced feeling uncomfortable or possibly even unhappy in one place of employment, while having felt very satisfied and comfortable in other work environments. There may be many reasons for these feelings, but the cultures of the different organisations and a personal reaction to them will have had a major influence on the experience.

To be comfortable and happy in a workplace, each person needs to understand the type of organisational culture, or cultures, that are possible. This understanding is critical to being able to operate and be efficient and effective in the workplace environment.

Types of organisational culture

There are four main types of organisational culture:

- power culture
- role culture
- task culture
- person culture.

The power culture

An organisation based on a power culture can best be described as a *web* (Fig 6-1). The success of this type of cultural organisation depends on a central power source that radiates out from the centre of the web. Around the centre of the web are the 'power rings'. The closer a ring is to the centre of the web the more powerful it is.

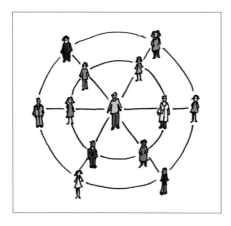

Fig 6-1 The power culture, represented by a web.

In the power culture, control over the organisation is governed by the individual in the centre and through a selection of key individuals – the power ring people – to implement the centre's policies. For example, a small dental practice may have a power culture, with the principal being at the centre of the web and the other team members forming the inner and outer power rings. It is the quality of the person at the centre of the web and that individual's ability to select team members to populate the rings of the web that is paramount to the success of the organisation.

There are few rules and procedures and little bureaucracy in a power culture. Control is exercised by the source of the power, the individual in the centre of the web, and implemented by the power ring members of the team. Strategy and direction is determined and dictated by the source of the power. The operation and development of the power culture is a top-down arrangement. In larger power culture organisations, the power source will, from time to time, 'venture out' across the web, supposedly to relate to others in the culture, but in reality to ascertain that strategy and direction are being followed.

The functioning of the power culture relies on the compliance and commitment of members of the team, rather than on meetings let alone personal initiative. As a consequence, team events in power cultures tend to be team briefings rather than interactive sessions. Understanding and acceptance of the wishes of the power source (the leader of the team), together with commitment to the aims and objectives of the organisation, are critical to the success of a power culture. When this type of culture works efficiently and effectively, the organisation tends to be proud and strong. If, however, the source of the power is inconsistent, or at any time weakened, hesitant or inconsistent, and, as a consequence, the power ring members are questioning or otherwise lacking conviction, the power culture web can be fragile and liable to disintegrate. In addition, size can be a problem for power cultures. A web can break down if its links or anchors are weak, or if it grows too big for the power source to control.

A power culture is threatened if the individual at the centre of the web changes. This may, for example, happen when the principal of a practice retires and a less dominant associate takes over control of the organisation. A change at the centre of the web will affect those individuals on the outer rings. There may be incompatibility or lack of trust in the new central power source. Under such circumstances, either the culture or the people in it have to change.

The role culture

The role culture is best seen as a Greek temple with strong supporting pillars representing different departments or other sections within the organisation (Fig 6-2). Those working in larger organisations such as a dental hospital or corporate dental body may work in a role culture. The centre of the organisation, the temple, is occupied by the governing body, surrounded by the pillars supporting the structure of the organisation. The pillars should be strong in their own right and able to function well both individually and collectively, with relatively little support from the central governing body. Provided that roles and responsibilities are fulfilled within the framework of the organisation, the role culture will be successful.

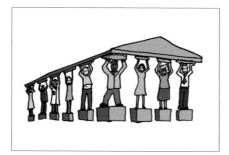

Fig 6-2 The role culture, represented by a Greek temple.

In the role culture, the roles and responsibilities of the members of the team are described, typically in the form of job descriptions. Having individuals perform satisfactorily, according to their job description and in compliance with the operational arrangements of the organisation underpins and reinforces the culture.

Role cultures offer security and predictability to the individual. It is generally the case, subject to satisfactory performance, that members of the dental team operating in successful role cultures have secure positions. The role culture may, however, prove frustrating to some individuals, who feel restricted by the arrangements governing the function of the culture. A role culture functions best when team working is optimal.

The task culture

The task culture is job or project orientated. It may be represented as a net, with the power being located at the intersections of the strands of the net (Fig 6-3). Some strands of the net may be thicker than others. Most of the power and influence lies at the major interstices—the knots of the net. The emphasis of the task culture is to get specific jobs done.

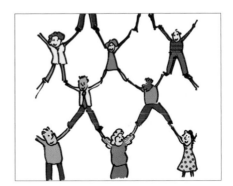

Fig 6-3 The task culture, represented by a net.

The task culture brings together the right people, at the right level and with the right resources and expects them to get on with specific tasks, ideally without the need to call on external support and guidance. The task culture is a team culture that utilises the power of the group to achieve its goals. Individuals have influence according to their expertise and standing in the team, rather than personal power. Individuals who succeed in task cultures have a high degree of control over their work.

The task culture is extremely adaptable. Groups or teams are formed for a specific purpose and can be reformed, disbanded or expanded according to changing circumstances. Individuals working in such a culture experience a high degree of control over their work; judgement is by results, and efficiency and effectiveness is highly dependent on interpersonal relationships and mutual respect amongst the members of the team. Standing in the team is based more on capacity and ability rather than age, experience or seniority.

Task cultures can run into difficulties when necessary resources are not available. This leads to low moral and frustration: a job to be done but not the wherewithal to do it. Under such circumstances, there is typically the need to change the culture and redeploy certain members of the team.

The person culture
The person culture is unusual. It can be visualised as a cluster or perhaps a galaxy of stars (Fig 6-4). In this culture, each individual is a focus of attention. Structure within a person culture organisation is minimal, if it exists at all.

Any structure formed is only there to serve the individuals within it. For example, a group of individuals, possible senior practitioners working in different practices or professors in a number of dental schools, could decide to work together as a group for individual and mutual benefit. The organisation within a person culture is very flat, with all those participating considering themselves to be of equal status, importance and influence. Organisations with this culture exist by mutual consent, without any form of hierarchy. Person cultures may be observed in such diverse situations as communes, large practices and university departments.

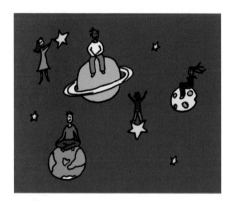

Fig 6-4 The person culture, represented by a galaxy of stars.

While it is unusual to find an organisation, especially within dentistry, where the person culture predominates, it is not unusual to find individuals whose personal preference is for this type of culture, but who find themselves having to work and operate in a different culture. For example, a professor is typically inclined towards a person culture but tends to work in a role culture. Specialists in organisations, for example consultants in hospitals or a specialist dental practitioner within a multisurgery practice, may try to behave as if they were part of a person culture and, as a consequence, lack allegiance to the organisation within which they work. Such behaviour can be very disruptive, if not damaging to the organisation. Individuals with this orientation are not easy to manage and may or may not be easy to work with.

Coexisting cultures
As in most workplace environments, more than one organisational culture may coexist. For example, in a large dental laboratory driven by a power or

role culture, people working within the different sections of the laboratory may be operating within a task culture. In other words, the head of a section of a dental laboratory may be the subject of a power or role culture, but the people working in the section may be a tight-knit team working on specific procedures or projects and, consequently, operating in a task culture. While everyone in the laboratory is working to achieve the same goal – high-quality laboratory work produced to a tight time schedule and on budget – there may be some conflict between the two organisational cultures, in particular, for the head of the section, who forms a bridge between the different cultures.

Finding a preferred cultural organisation

The characteristics of the various organisational cultures are summarised in Table 6-1. Different people will be happy and successful in one culture, but not in another. It follows, therefore, that for professional success and personal happiness an individual should strive to find employment, or to develop a culture that matches their preference.

Table 6-1 **Summary of organisational cultures**

Power culture	Role culture	Task culture	Person culture
Informal	Formal	Team approach	Mutual consent
Central control	Prescriptive	Task oriented	No hierarchy
Reluctance to change	Security	Little interference	Too idealistic for general practice
Quality of centre paramount	Bureaucracy	Could change to power culture	Voluntary organisations

Understanding one's own preferences for organising culture should make it easier to decide which type of culture best suits both personal and professional needs. First, we need to identify in which culture we function best: one with rigorous rules and protocols, or one with a more laid-back approach to leadership. Do we prefer to be left to our own devices, as long as we achieve the team objective, or do we want strict control from others, so we know where we stand?

69

When these questions have been answered, it becomes possible to consider the type of cultural organisation will make us feel most happy. The beauty of working within the dental profession is that there is such a variety of career opportunities that it should be possible to join, or develop an organisational culture in which to flourish and realise personal goals.

Working in a power culture

The traditional dental practice will most often have a power culture, with the principal of the practice at the centre of the 'web'. As described above, certain power will be delegated to key individuals, such as the practice manager or the senior dental nurse to ensure the smooth running of the practice.

Everything will run smoothly as long as the individuals think the same way, or accept the thinking of the central person. This type of culture can suit individuals who view their team role as team workers, who are compliant, who can accept strong, possibly dominant leadership, and who understand that the team leader, typically the principal in general dental practice, thrives on the pressures associated with owning the practice.

It is important to remember that harmony and, in turn, the success of the power culture web is largely dependent on the personality and leadership qualities of the person occupying the centre. An ideal web culture relies on common acceptance of the organisational philosophy. If the person at the centre is weak, inconsistent, or a poor communicator, then the individuals on the web—the members of the team and particularly those on the outer rings—can feel ignored or undervalued and so become frustrated. In such circumstances, there can be negative feelings and disincentives to efficiency and effectiveness in the culture, which may, in certain cases break down.

Working in a role culture

A corporate dental practice or dental hospital tends to differ from the traditional practice in having a hierarchal structure and typically rigorous protocols on, for example, aspects of personal behaviour and treatment of patients. Corporate dentistry and dental hospitals invariably adopt the role culture, with its prescriptive ethos applying equally to all members of the team. The members of the senior management of the organisation occupy the centre of the role culture 'temple', managing and otherwise controlling the various sections or departments of the organisation, which form the pillars of the culture.

This type of environment suits individuals who want to work in an organisation in which they know where they stand and can accept, possibly even find comfort in, the rigid rules and regulations that apply to everyone in the organisation.

Individuals who view their team role as implementers may work well in this culture, as it is likely to appeal to their disciplined and reliable nature, particularly if the individuals they are working with are similarly minded. Individuals ill-suited to operating in a role culture, but finding themselves working in such an organisation, can feel restricted by the prescriptive nature of the rules and protocols and, as a consequence, challenged both in terms of personal autonomy and in opportunity to innovate, let alone make small changes to processes and procedures.

Working in a task culture
The organisation with a task culture appeals to individuals who prefer to specialise in specific areas and wish to practice their skill with as little influence as possible from other individuals. For example, a dental technician may have a flair for a certain aspect of dental technology and a wish to work in an environment and culture in which it is possible to further develop these particular skills. In this environment, tasks are likely to be assigned and coordinated by a third person.

The task culture best suits individuals who are team workers who can provide mutual support for each other. It also suits those who see their role as specialist.

The task culture does not appeal to the individual who dislikes doing repetitive work and is constantly seeking to broaden their horizons.

Working in a person culture
A person culture appeals to individuals who like a large degree of autonomy and freely volunteer their skills and expertise to help others. This type of organisation has little hierarchy given its reliance on the altruism of the individuals within it.

This culture may arguably thrive only when everyone in the team sees their role as a team player. Such cultures may be at risk of poor efficiency and effectiveness given lack of clear leadership, structure and organisation.

Conclusions

Historically, individuals within organisations were likened to machines that could be controlled. Thinking has moved on to view individuals in organisations as collections of people who can contribute to a productive workplace, assuming control within the organisation is fair and effective.

Any individual who has chosen a career in dentistry has the opportunity to experience working in a wide range of organisational cultures and to choose the organisation type that best serves their own personal well-being and career goals. If members of the dental team feel frustrated and trapped in their present organisation/work culture, consideration should be given to a new career direction, or possibly just a change of role within the existing organisation.

Further reading

Belbin RM. Team Roles at Work. London: Butterworth-Heinemann, 2004.

Handy C. Understanding Organisations, 4th edn. London: Penguin, 1999.

Chapter 7
Team roles and responsibilities

Carole Brennan and Marina Harris

Aim

The aim of this chapter is to describe the behaviour of individuals in terms of team roles and how the various dental team members interact with each other in the workplace.

Outcome

The chapter should lead to an understanding of the commonly identified roles that people play in teams and appreciate that some team roles complement each other better than others. Readers should also be able to analyse the balance of the team roles that exist in their own place of work.

Introduction

Research into the behaviour of individuals as part of a team indicates that people take on particular roles in teams, and that it is the balance of these roles which determines the success of the team.

> The composition of a team, and the ways in which the team members complement each other, is critical to success.

What is a team role?

The term team role refers to behaving, contributing and interrelating with others in the workplace and related environments in a mutually beneficial way. For practical purposes, it is necessary to distinguish between an individual's team role and their functional role. A person's functional role is the specific functions they perform, but their team role may, for example, be leader, coordinator or implementer.

Individuals in a team with similar functional roles are likely to vary greatly in their team role. For example, the functional role of dental nurses working in the same dental practice will, in all probability, be exactly the same, but their team role may vary greatly to best meet the needs of the practice.

Factors in team role behaviour

The ways in which we come to behave as we do are complex and beyond the scope of this book. A simple schematic of factors influencing behaviour is reproduced in Fig 7-1.

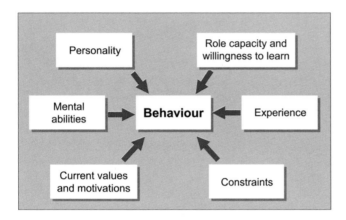

Fig 7-1
Simple schematic of factors influencing team behaviour.

These factors can be enlarged upon:

→ *personality:* psychophysiological factors, such as extroversion or introversion, and high or low anxiety traits affecting behaviour
→ *mental abilities:* high-level thinking and mental agility, which can override negative personality traits to encourage favourable behaviours
→ *current values and motivations:* personal ways of seeing yourself
→ *constraints:* factors in the immediate environment which influence behaviour, for example feeling awkward and shy in the presence of senior members of the team
→ *experience:* the accumulation of experience in life, which tempers behaviour
→ *capacity and willingness to learn:* learning about roles of others and being able to appreciate variations in personality and, in turn, behaviours.

Simply put, individuals tend to adopt a stable pattern of association with other members of their team. This is based on personality, which is modified by the thought process, and then further modified by personal values, governed by perceived constraints, influenced by experience and added to by sophisticated learning.

Types of team role

The types of behaviour that people engage in are infinite, but the range of behaviours that make an effective contribution to a team's performance can be narrowed down to nine team roles (Table 7-1). These roles all have their strengths and weaknesses.

Strengths and weaknesses

The more prominent the strengths of an individual, the more conspicuous the weaknesses can be. That is why powerful individuals may be as renowned for their quirks as for their talents. Allowable weaknesses are those weaknesses that emphasise strengths.

Do weaknesses matter? If the weaknesses are the price to be paid for important strengths, and other members of the team can compensate for the individual's weakness, then it may be a small price to pay.

Allowable weaknesses should generally be accepted and not corrected, because such correction could undermine the strengths of the individual. There is, however, a fine line between allowable weaknesses and unacceptable behaviour. These differences are outlined in Table 7-2.

Who is occupying which role?

It is a useful exercise to consider some of the following suggestions to see if you can identify, first, your own team role and, second the roles of your colleagues. It may not be that easy to categorise oneself or others into one defined role. Generally, an individual will have a strong leaning towards one role, but have some characteristics of one or more other roles. Getting a group of colleagues to categorise themselves can stimulate some interesting discussion. Do you all see the same things in each other? How do your colleagues see you?

There are a number of benefits in this exercise.

Table 7-1 **Types of team role and allowable weaknesses**

Role	Strengths	Allowable weaknesses
Plant	Creative, imaginative and unorthodox; solves difficult problems	Ignores details; too preoccupied to communicate effectively
Resource investigator	Extrovert, enthusiastic, communicative; explores opportunities and develops contacts	Overoptimistic; loses interest once initial enthusiasm has passed
Coordinator	Mature, confident, a good chairperson; clarifies goals, promotes decision making and delegates effectively	Can be seen as wily and manipulative
Shaper	Challenging, dynamic, thrives on pressure; has the drive and courage to overcome obstacles	Can provoke others, possibly hurting their feelings
Monitor evaluator	Sober, strategic and discerning; sees all options and tends to judge accurately	Lacks drive and ability to inspire others; may be overly critical
Team worker	Cooperative, mild, perceptive and diplomatic; listens, builds, avoids friction and has a calming influence	Indecisive in difficult situations; can be easily influenced
Implementer	Disciplined, reliable, conservative and efficient; turns ideas into practical actions	Somewhat inflexible, slow to respond to new possibilities
Completer	Painstaking, conscientious and anxious; searches out errors and omissions but delivers on time	Inclined to worry unduly; reluctant to delegate and tends to be overly concerned with detail
Specialist	Single minded, self-starting, and dedicated; provides knowledge and special skills	Contributes on a narrow front; dwells on technicalities, overlooking the 'big picture'

Table 7-2 **Team roles and allowable and unacceptable weaknesses**

Team role	Allowable weakness	Unacceptable weakness
Plant	Preoccupation with ideas and neglect of practical matters	Strong 'ownership' of idea when cooperation with others would yield better results
Resource investigator	Loss of enthusiasm once initial excitement has passed	Letting clients/patients or colleagues down by neglecting to follow up arrangements
Coordinator	An inclination to be lazy if someone else can be found to do the work	Taking credit for the team effort
Shaper	A proneness to frustration and irritation	Inability to recover a situation with good humour or apology
Monitor evaluator	Scepticism with logic	Cynicism without logic
Team worker	Indecision on crucial issues	Avoiding situations that may entail pressure
Implementer	Adherence to the orthodox and proven	Obstructing change
Completer	Perfectionism	Obsessive behaviour
Specialist	Acquiring knowledge for its own sake	Ignoring factors outside own area of competence

- You will be better able to understand how and why you all get on, or otherwise, as the case may be. With this increased understanding comes an increased tolerance of the behaviour of colleagues, even if it is somewhat irritating.
- You will be able to analyse the balance of the team in which you work. If you are fortunate, you will work with colleagues who complement each other. Or, you might discover that your team is top heavy with shapers and plants, with not enough team workers or resource investigators to smooth the way.

- If you identify that you are part of a dysfunctional team, it may not be a problem as long as you are happy at work and you and the team are accomplishing agreed goals. If, however, you find that you are not enjoying your work and feel stressed or anxious, then you may need to consider if it is in your best interests to remain part of that team.
- It is always worth recognising your own strengths and weakness, in particular, when it comes to interviews and appraisals. This helps to promote positive discussion in respect of your personal development.

Interpersonal chemistry in the workplace

When working as part of a dental team, which, more often than not, will involve dynamic interpersonal relationships, the range of different individuals (team roles) will influence the way in which people will react to each other. For example, if a shaper displays aggression at work, team workers may react by using their calming influence. If, however, the situation arises when a shaper displays aggression to another shaper, an argument may ensue—a personality clash.

There are a number of possible interpersonal reactions at work, which can affect the three main status levels: the boss, the peer group and subordinates.

Shaper relationships

Shapers can present particular problems in some working relationships. On the asset side, they are achievers. They are more likely to gain promotion and force themselves up to the top than any other team role group. On the debit side, some organisations run by shapers are subject to crises—rows, poor industrial relationships and fracture of the team.

→ *With the boss.* Shapers are most happy working with a boss who does not interfere, but will give advice as and when needed. Monitor evaluators can make effective bosses of shapers so long as they are respected. Coordinator bosses possess the people skills to cope effectively with all but the most difficult of shapers. A boss who is an implementer does not like the risk of the disturbance a shaper subordinate is likely to bring to a well-ordered system.
→ *With peers.* Shapers prefer colleagues who are dynamic, such as resource investigators. A colleague who is a plant would view the cut and thrust of the shaper as a threat to the plant's creative role in the team.
→ *With subordinates.* Shaper bosses like team workers who can deal with the dominance of a shaper boss, and who may even be able to manipulate the

boss with discretion. Implementers also make good subordinates. A competer can serve a shaper boss well, but there is always the prospect of the inevitable tension becoming too great. The relationships of a shaper boss with coordinators and monitor evaluators are less satisfactory, given the possibility of clash of style.

Plant relationships
The plant can be preoccupied and can find practical issues and cooperation difficult to achieve.

→ *With the boss.* The ideal boss for a plant is a coordinator who is good at discovering talent and knowing where and when to use it. A sympathetic and supportive team worker boss can also bring out the best in a plant. At the other end of the scale, shapers and implementers as bosses are likely to show the greatest intolerance towards plants.

→ *With peers.* Plants can make stimulating colleagues and associate well with the sociable coordinators, resource investigators and team workers. Plants clash with monitor evaluators and other plants—even though they are drawn towards each other. Plants most risk clashing with implementers as their basic aims and values have little in common.

→ *With subordinates.* In contrast to the relationship with peers, the plant boss has a very good relationship with an implementer subordinate. Whatever differences in outlook occur, the plant boss–implementer subordinate relationship is one of the most effective, if it can be established. The plant boss realises that an implementer will act upon an idea, if it is judged practical. Another valued relationship is with the monitor evaluator as a subordinate. As colleagues they would argue, but with the difference in status the plant is more confident in proposing ideas or suggestions. Plants, who tend to be preoccupied, are least happy with resource investigators and shapers as subordinates, given their cut and thrust nature, which can challenge the sensitivity of a boss who is a plant.

Specialist relationships
Specialists take a pride in their work and in controlling their activities. They can do without bosses, colleagues or subordinates. In reality, specialists have to deal with others since 'no man is an island'.

→ *With the boss.* Specialists need a boss who believes in and values their expertise and will give them a loose rein. Specialists respond well to team workers and coordinators, who believe in a delegation of responsibility. The opposite situation applies to resource investigators and shapers as they do not accept the specialist as being self-governing, and they will intrude. The specialist will view this intrusion negatively.

→ *With peers.* Specialists appear to work best with implementers and team workers, through mutual respect. But it is a different matter when it comes to plants. Plants see every problem as a challenge, and it matters little if that problem resides in the specialist's territory. In the peer group, conflicts of this nature are not easily resolved.

→ *With subordinates.* A specialist boss likes subordinates to treat them with respect. Implementers and team workers make good subordinates. Once again, the plants pose a problem; as they prefer lateral thinking rather than observance of established standards, their conduct is liable to be interpreted as insubordination.

Monitor evaluator relationships
One major consideration, underlying all others, is that monitor evaluators generally keep a low profile and, as a consequence, need to be discovered if they are to be able to contribute fully to the team.

→ *With the boss.* Monitor evaluators work best for a coordinator boss, who consults and seeks advice. A shaper boss would be too bold and decisive for a monitor evaluator's liking.

→ *With peers.* Monitor evaluators prefer coordinators and implementers who liaise well. They work least well with other monitor evaluators or completers, who tend to go into lengthy debate over relatively trivial matters, causing delay and uncertainty.

→ *With subordinates.* Implementers make best subordinates because of their efficiency in devising methods and supervising their work. Monitor evaluators do not usually clash with their subordinate, but should avoid other monitor evaluators and plants, given their tendency to deliberate, leading to inaction.

Completer relationships
Completers are perfectionists in nature and need to ensure accurate delivery on time; this leads to a tendency to become overly concerned with controlling all the details themselves.

→ *With the boss.* The aptitude of completers for following through a job and getting results makes them good subordinates for bosses who are keen initiators and value results. Completers work well for resource investigators, plants and shapers. They perform less well when they report to a boss who also a completer, as such a relationship can result in tension.

→ *With peers.* Completers are respected most by implementers, as they share the same style and values. They clash with resource investigators, who see the completer as fussy and restricted, in contrast to the completer seeing the resource investigator as careless and erratic.

→ *With subordinates.* As in the peer group, completers, who tend to worry unduly, like implementers as subordinates because they are well organised and reliable. They are least well disposed towards resource implementers.

Implementer relationships

Since implementers have an exceptional readiness to address the practical demands of situations, systems and organisations, they work well with a broad cross-section of people, both as bosses and colleagues. But when relationships do go wrong, they can go badly wrong.

→ *With the boss.* Implementers prefer bosses who look for good organisation skills, such as shapers and plants. Implementers also work well for the completer boss, who values efficient follow through. Relationships are generally less successful if the boss is also an implementer, as this often leads to increased bureaucracy.

→ *With peers.* Implementers work well with coordinators, monitor evaluators, resource investigators, completers and specialists. Generally, implementers work well with a broad cross-section of people.

→ *With subordinates.* Implementers tend to develop a more formal relationship with their subordinates. Compliant team workers suit them best. Implementers find plants and resource investigators the most difficult type of subordinates to work with, given their lack of respect for authority.

Resource investigator relationships

Resource investigators, being sociable and generally tolerant, are not too fussy about the nature of their work colleagues.

→ *With the boss.* Resource investigators cope well with shaper bosses because they can stand up to the pressures and hold their own. They do, however, dislike completer and specialist bosses, who value precision and keep a short rein on their subordinates.

→ *With peers.* Resource investigators work well with implementers and team workers, where they can establish cooperation. They do not work well with completers and specialists, given their irreconcilable differences in style.

→ *With subordinates.* Completers make good subordinates because they compensate for the weaknesses of the typical resource investigators behaviour, notably dashing around and leaving a trail of unfinished work behind them. Resource investigators are happy to work with a wide range of subordinates, but relationships may not always be effective. The danger is that subordinates may sit around wasting time, as the resource investigator has not found time to give them instructions.

Coordinator relationships
Coordinators are usually adept at handling personal relationships and can cope with giving orders, as well as receiving them. Coordinators also deal well with talented people.

→ *With the boss.* Coordinators are amongst the most effective in relating to shaper bosses; they will do the job, but will also stand up to the boss if necessary. Coordinators also make their mark with plant bosses. Coordinators are less keen on working for team worker bosses, given that there may be a severe lack of direction.

→ *With peers.* Coordinators work especially well with team workers on the social front and with implementers on the organisation front. They clash with shapers.

→ *With subordinates.* Coordinators make good supervisors. Their talents are especially marked in managing plants, as clever, creative people can be difficult to manage. A shaper subordinate is likely to challenge the style and decisions of a coordinator boss.

Team worker relationships
Team workers are amongst the easiest people to work with. Any dangers that may arise are more likely to relate to effectiveness than to matters of compatibility.

→ *With the boss.* Ideally team workers should report to a strong shaper boss to encourage drive and challenge and, conversely, should avoid a team worker boss, whose decisiveness may be held in question.

→ *With peers.* Team workers work especially well with other team workers, providing mutual support for each other. They also act as good colleagues for plants. Shaper colleagues can sometimes unsettle team workers in their desire for advancement in the organisation.

→ *With subordinates.* Team worker bosses like self-assured subordinates who also pose no threat to their authority. Shapers are seen as a challenge and will put pressure on a team worker boss.

Conclusions

Dental healthcare professionals mostly occupy a team role within a dental team. Some teams will be more successful than others. Some teams will be cohesive, others fragmented. This may relate to the balance of team roles at the three working levels: the boss, peers and subordinates. The composition of a team and the ways in which the members of the team complement each other is critical to the success of the team.

Further reading

Belbin RM. Team Roles at Work. London: Butterworth-Heinemann, 2004.

Chapter 8
Efficiency and effectiveness

Carole Brennan

Aim

The aim of this chapter is to help the dental team to make best use of time, reduce stress levels, perform well at work and achieve goals.

Outcome

After reading this chapter, readers should appreciate that time is valuable and easily wasted and recognise how time is spent and how to prioritise tasks. There should also be awareness that good time management reduces stress levels and that strategies can be developed to enhance efficiency and effectiveness.

Time

Time cannot be bought, borrowed or manufactured, so there is only ever 60 seconds in a minute, 60 minutes in an hour and 24 hours in a day. Time spent (or wasted) is gone and cannot be retrieved.

The 24 hours in each person's day is the same as that in everybody else's day (Fig 8-1), and yet often one can end up feeling short of time, tired, angry, frustrated and stressed. Could it be that you are not using, or do not know how to use, the 24 hours to best advantage? Alternatively, are you unrealistic as to what can be achieved in a day?

Time management refers to the process of actively structuring time in ways that enable the individual to be more productive, with less stress and with increased probability of achieving professional and personal goals.

In the fast-moving society in which we live, we work harder, longer and faster and often with less support than ever before. Mastering time management is not an option, but an essential survival skill in high-pressure situations such as those that exist in busy practices and other clinical environments.

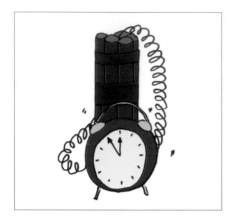

Fig 8-1 Time needs management.

Time can be classified in various ways. In the context of efficiency and effectiveness, time may be considered under the following headings.

→ *Time to sell.* This is the time which is given over to running a business, sold to an employer or as students given to school, college or university. The pay-off is remuneration, skills, occupational qualifications or education. Sold time goes typically well beyond actual hours worked; it also includes, for example, time spent travelling and working at home.
→ *Maintenance time.* This is time used to keep things ticking over; time spent in individual maintenance: eating, sleeping, dealing with personal affairs, looking after others and a home.
→ *Time to choose.* This is the time left over, which is free to be used to pursue interests and relax.

Finding the time

Many of us feel that we do not 'have the time'. How many times have we heard ourselves, friends and colleagues say: 'I haven't had the time to do that yet'. In a profession such as dentistry, whatever the personal goals in life, an individual needs to perform well at work and to create a work–life balance that is sustainable.

The consequences of a work–life balance that is unsustainable, if not out of control, include stress, ill-health, not achieving the things that are important to you, poor performance, neglecting family and friends and not having the time to relax and enjoy life.

Managing time well

To address personal time management, answer 'true' or 'false' to the following statements:

1. I never seem to have enough time for things
2. I rarely get things done on time
3. I can always find time for myself
4. I always know what I'm doing and why
5. I keep lists of things I need to do
6. I plan my day by setting objectives and priorities.

A person who has learnt to manage time well should be able to answer:

1. False
2. False
3. True
4. True
5. True
6. True.

If your answers were different, even if only in one or two of the questions, then there is a need to develop, or at least improve, your time management skills.

The first step in time management is to know how you are currently spending your time. Once you have a clear picture of this, you can begin to take control of it and start to redirect your time usage towards your goals and their priorities

Current use of time

There are a number of techniques for analysing how time is being spent. These include activity logs and time management grids, which are discussed below.

Activity logs

Activity logs help you to analyse how you actually spend your time. The first time you use an activity log, you may be shocked to discover how much time you waste or put to no good use.

It is necessary to go through the process of writing everything down, as memory and subjective judgement are a poor substitute for objective data. Keeping an activity log for several days helps you to understand how you actually spend your time, and to identify the times of the day when you perform best.

Completing and analysing your activity log will help you to identify the reasons why, for example, you are always working through lunch, staying late in the evening, not achieving your goals or working on too many things at any one time. Furthermore, you can identify the reasons for your endless 'busyness'. Is it poor organisation? Is it outdated or malfunctioning equipment that is constantly affecting the smooth running of your day? When you understand who or what is wasting your time, you can take action to regain control of your time management.

It is also important to record in your activity log how you feel at different times, whether alert, flat, tired or energetic, and how much you obtained satisfaction or begrudged doing particular tasks.

With the analysis of your activity log completed, identify time wasted, time doing tasks that were important and necessary, time spent doing tasks that could have waited or been done by someone else, and time spent doing other things.

Once you know how you spent your time, answer the following questions.

- Does anything surprise you about the way you have spent the last few days?
- Was there anything unusual about the last few days?
- What returns are you getting for your time investment: satisfaction, peace of mind, remuneration?
- Are there any changes you would like to make?
- Can you identify ways of saving time, to enhance and ideally maximise your returns?
- Is it necessary to critically review what you expect to achieve in the time available?

Establishing priorities
Having analysed your activity log and answered the questions above, you need to consider the amount of energy you spend on various tasks and whether those tasks justify the effort expended.

Many people spend their days in a frenzy of activity but achieve very little through lack of appreciation and focus on the most important things. Vilfedo Pareto, an Italian economist, developed what is often referred to as the 'Pareto Principle', or the '80/20 rule'. This states that typically 80% of unfocused effort generates only 20% of results, with the remaining 80% of results being achieved with 20% of focused effort.

In other words, much more can be achieved by increasing the extent to which your efforts are focused.

Time management grid

The time management grid (Fig 8-2) is a useful tool in helping to sort out priorities.

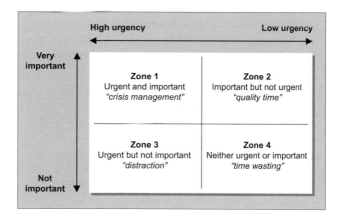

Fig 8-2 Time management grid.

The time management grid focuses on the two key elements of time management: the *urgency* and the *importance* of tasks. Along the top of the grid is the urgency axis: the left-hand side of the axis is very urgent and the right-hand side is less urgent. The vertical axis of the grid is the importance axis. The top boxes contain more important activities; the bottom boxes contain activities that are less important. This gives four time zones.

→ *Zone 1.* This represents things that are both urgent and important, or in other words things requiring 'crisis management'. These activities must be dealt with immediately. There are times when a crisis occurs which cannot be predicted, or the circumstances for their occurrence are out of your control, for example a medical emergency. All planned work has to be abandoned to manage the crisis. There are times when a task becomes a crisis simply because it was not allocated the appropriate time or priority and dealt with accordingly in a timely fashion.

→ *Zone 2.* This represents things that are important but not urgent. Termed 'quality time', the activities in this quadrant are important but do not have to be done immediately. The type of things that should appear in this box includes routine tasks, maintenance procedures and regular events. Activities that appear in this box are important, and time and energy are required to cope with them in a timely, effective manner. These tasks are best done at the time of the day when there is the least risk of disruption.

→ *Zone 3.* These are the distractions. They must be dealt with as they occur but are often of little, if any, consequence. Typical distractions include unsolicited telephone calls and chatting to colleagues over trivial, inconsequential matters.

→ *Zone 4.* The time wasters sit in zone 4. These are things that are neither urgent nor important. Examples include reading junk mail, day dreaming and doing inconsequential tasks that should be done by someone else, if at all.

> Putting off things which should be done today is the making of a crisis tomorrow.

Using the time management grid

Using the information obtained from your activity log, identify what proportions of the day are spent in the different zones of the time management grid.

You should spend as little time as possible on zone 1 activities. Spending your days coping with one crisis after another is extremely stressful and inefficient, eating up the time required to deal with other important tasks, which, if left unattended, will become tomorrow's crisis.

Ideally, a good proportion of your time should be spent in zone 2. This is time spent doing important tasks in a timely manner, enabling you to perform well at work and achieve your goals. Because zone 2 tasks are important, they should be scheduled to be completed when you are most alert and productive. If you are a 'morning person', allocate time to deal with these tasks in the morning, ideally leaving time for other tasks in the afternoon when your energy and attention levels are lower.

If you find that you spend too much of your day in zone 3, constantly being distracted, you may feel that you have been busy all day but have not really achieved anything. Under such circumstances, action is required to reduce or eliminate the distractions.

How much of your day is spent in zone 4? A small proportion of time in this zone is inevitable, possibly even important, but too much time wasted is a sign of an urgent need to review your priorities. Some people like to be in zone 4 – busy doing nothing, putting off tackling 'harder tasks'. Zone 4 activities are best planned when your concentration is low and you are beginning to wane, typically at the end of the day.

Taking control of your time

Once you have a clear picture of how you are currently using your time, you can begin to take control of this important resource. The foundation of managing your time is a firm understanding of your goals and their priorities.

Identifying goals

Many people have, at any one time, no more than a general idea of what they want to achieve at work and in their personal life. To make better use of time, it is important to become more goal orientated and to:

- become more aware of what you are trying to achieve in your key roles and other aspects of your life, in both the short and longer term
- make a plan; this may involve annual, quarterly, monthly, weekly or possibly even daily planning
- recognise and prioritise not only the tasks that you have to do, but also the things that you want to do.

If goals, plans and priorities are not committed to paper, then it is all too easy to let them slip. Committing to paper, possibly including timeframes, involves resolve and determination, let alone the possibility of facing and making decisions about life in general. It is so much harder to throw away a piece of paper summarising your aspiration than to quietly forget a list in your mind.

When setting goals, remember the acronym SMART. Goals should be:

→ *Specific.* This means having clearly defined goals; make sure you identify exactly want you want to achieve, particularly before spending time and effort in achieving goals you consider unimportant.

→ *Measurable.* There must be some way of measuring how far you have gone and how far you need to go to achieve your goals. Honesty in self-assessment can be difficult.

→ *Agreed upon.* This means that you and others involved or affected are of a similar opinion and will be supportive of each other.

→ *Reachable.* The goal must be achievable.

→ *Timed.* Have a timeframe. Know when the goal must be started and finished.

Be SMART.

Establishing priorities

Once you have set your goals, they need to be prioritised: those which should be tackled first, those which can be delayed and those to follow. You can then plan your activities to focus on furthering your goals, instead of getting hopelessly sidetracked by distractions and other diversions.

Planning use of time

Once it is clear what the goals and priorities are, the next step is to plan time usage to enable these to be fulfilled. There are a number of ways to do this.

Planning grids

Planning grids are one of the best tools for organising workload and making sure that routine tasks and goals are completed on time. Start with an annual grid. This may be a calendar, diary, electronic personnel organiser or a computer software programme. After developing an annual schedule, prepare a monthly calendar, transferring important dates and deadlines, then breakdown tasks into a weekly schedule, identifying priorities and the time required to complete them. Once the week ahead is planned, it is now possible to begin to organise the day.

Remember:

- create a favourable work–life balance; the focus is on achieving results, not being busy
- distribute the time to be spent each day in the various time zones in the time management grid (Fig 8-2)
- revisit the weekly, monthly and annual plan on a regular basis to adjust and refine according to changing circumstances.

Making lists

Many people find a 'to-do' list to be a useful tool in successful time management. A reluctance to commit to preparing to-do lists may be a symptom of a failure to get to grips with time management. The advantages of making a list, rather than relying on memory, include:

- ensures that items are not forgotten
- makes prioritisation more effective
- reinforces commitment.

Different people use to-do lists in different ways in different situations, but consider the following suggestions.

- Motivation is enhanced by keeping lists short, with the aim of completing a list on a daily basis.
- Some goals and tasks are complex and dependent on other people; these should be broken down to component parts to allow them to be 'chipped away' on a daily basis moving towards the overall objective.
- Colour coding or otherwise classifying lists helps prioritising and improves the sense of achievement: for example, red to underline things that must be done today, green for things that should be completed today and blue for things that would be a bonus to achieve. As each task is completed, it is crossed off the list. This supports a sense of achievement at the end of the day, seeing a set of red and other items crossed off the list.
- Keep in mind that even the best tools for time management can become a task in themselves. Making a list and using it each day is a powerful tool, but if several lists are being compiled each day then the focus may become the lists rather than the tasks they include.
- According to individual ways of working and circumstances, weekly lists or possibly even perpetual, rolling lists may be more motivating than daily lists.

Whatever approach is adopted, a to-do list should encourage steady progress towards goals being achieved.

Eliminating time wasting

Many people are aware that a degree of their time is wasted, but are unaware of the extent of the problem and the reasons why it happens, and, most importantly, lack the knowledge or skills to reduce or control the amount of time being wasted.

Procrastination and distraction are among the most common 'time wasters', and these are discussed below together with suggestions for coping with them.

Procrastination (negative delay)
Procrastination masquerades in numerous disguises. Putting things off until tomorrow that could or should be done today invariably wastes time. Procrastination is a form of negative delay; it slows down achievement and restricts future opportunities. Procrastination also tends to have a domino effect: what should be done tomorrow has to be delayed to do what should have been done today.

> Procrastination is the thief of time (Edward Young 1683–1765).

Procrastination presents in a number of ways.

→ *Overplanning.* Some people waste time over planning, possibly to avoid getting on with the tasks in hand. Contingency planning has its place, but should be linked to the risk of primary plans failing.
→ *Perfectionism.* Perfectionists waste time fussing over details when tasks have been successfully achieved. This delays tackling other problems. Often perfectionism is not required and is not cost-effective. Most people strive to complete tasks to the best of their ability, but there are occasions when circumstances dictate a degree of pragmatism. Knowing when to stop and move on can be a great time saver.
→ *Boredom.* Boring jobs are very easy to delay for spurious reasons. Here self-discipline is needed. Set specific times for the boring jobs, preferably at or near the beginning of the day, with the prospect of moving on to more enjoyable tasks.
→ *Hostility.* If there is hostility towards a task, or the person giving the task, there is a strong temptation to delay. Delay, however, tends to aggravate hostility, with the potential for distraction and all more wastage of time.
→ *The deadline high.* Coming up against a tight deadline and meeting it is immensely satisfying. It can be associated with strong rushes of adrenaline. The problems with this are that tasks may end up being rushed and not completed satisfactorily and deadlines may be missed if there are any last minute complications. Deadline highs are stress related.

Positive delay
Occasionally delay can be positive and useful:

• when tired, upset or angry, it is often best not to tackle jobs that require sensitivity and clarity of thought
• when the information or understanding to do the job properly is not available, it is best to delay until these are acquired
• when matters may be resolved by other means in the intervening period, a delay can be considered 'masterly inactivity'

The positive aspects of delay must not, however, be used as an excuse to avoid action that is obvious and necessary.

Distractions
Whatever approach is adopted to time management, it is inevitable that a number of distractions will be encountered. Minor delays and distractions add up to a major source of time wasting, and these need to be identified and strategies developed for dealing with them. Some common distractions are sidelining issues, telephone calls and visitors.

→ *Sidelining issues.* This includes unnecessary time spent surfing the net and getting involved in other people's business and affairs. If you know you have a tendency to let time run away with you, then consider controlling this tendency through self-discipline, particularly when there are pressing issues awaiting your attention.
→ *Unwanted telephone calls.* These may be work or family and friends related. If they distract you from completing important tasks, let casual callers know that you cannot speak to them at present and suggest a time when you could call back. When dealing with pressing issues, turn on the answer phone and deal with messages at a more convenient time.
→ *Unwanted visitors.* To avoid distractions from unwanted (unscheduled) visitors, let people know that you do not want to be interrupted. Close the door to your work environment and, if necessary, put up a 'do not disturb' sign.

Learning to delegate
The ability and willingness to delegate is central to good time management.

Analysing an activity log can identify just how much of your time is spent doing tasks that could and, importantly, should be done by someone else. There are several common reasons for failing to delegate.

95

- You may be reluctant to hand over certain tasks because you have always done them, you do them easily and you do them well. What's more, they are often the jobs that you enjoy.
- Work and responsibilities have a way of expanding, sometimes so imperceptibly that you fail to notice it happening. Also, as you become more experienced and competent at work and take on more responsibilities, the delegation of tasks that no longer are required to be done by you personally is often overlooked.
- If you hold the belief that the only way to get a job done properly is to do it yourself, you will never completely master the art of delegation and, in turn, effective time management.

Learning to say 'No'

For many, the inability to say 'No' is largely responsible for being too busy. It is possible to learn say 'No' in an appropriate and confident manner that will not result in conflict or confrontation. Indeed, being able to say 'No' at appropriate times can strengthen a person's position and standing.

Decluttering the working environment

Having a tidy organised working environment undoubtedly saves time, reduces stress levels and increases effectiveness (Fig 8-3). An efficient filing system and a tidy desk will help in processing work smoothly, allowing access to information in seconds rather than spending minutes searching through heaps of papers.

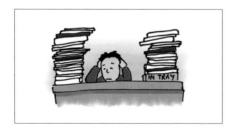

Fig 8-3 The cluttered desk overwhelms the best of intentions.

In a laboratory or surgery environment, tidiness is important not just for increased efficiency and effectiveness but also for infection control and health and safety.

Remembering to relax

Once you have gained control over your use of time, you will have the time to relate to colleagues and you will have time to do things you want to and enjoy doing. In this way, you should be more efficient, effective and approachable, while appearing relaxed and in control: a goal worth striving for in an environment in which there are ever increasing pressures on individuals and their time.

Finally, Box 8-1 lists some quick and easy time tips.

Make an effort to get satisfaction out of everything you do
Find something to enjoy in whatever you do
Stop regretting your failures and learn from your mistakes
Remind yourself that there is always enough time for important things
Continually look at ways of freeing up your time
Examine the ways you have always done things; is it still the most efficient way?
Use waiting time to relax, make notes and review lists
Keep your long-term goals in mind and review your progress towards them
Look ahead in your month and try to anticipate what is going to happen so you can better schedule your time
Reward yourself for getting things done on time
Have confidence in yourself and in your judgement of priorities and stick to them
Do first things first
When you catch yourself procrastinating, ask yourself what you are avoiding
Put your efforts into areas that provide long-term benefits
Push yourself and be persistent when you know you are doing well
Think on paper when possible – it makes it easier to review and revise
Seek help and ask for advice when needed

Conclusions

At the heart of good time management is the shift of focus to *concentrating on results, not on being busy*. Good time management is one of the core differences between effective and ineffective people.

Everyone needs to set priorities, both for the short and the long term. It is all too easy to slide along doing what is easiest, or doing what other people would have you do and what is habitual. It is also easy to fall into the trap of letting others spend your time for you, when you should be concentrating on doing what will bring you the best returns.

Manage time by:

- using an activity log to evaluate use of time
- knowing how much your time is worth
- determining what is important for success in your job, and what constitutes exceptional performance
- setting goals and plans that will lead to success.

Use time effectively by:

- doing important work in quality time
- spending more time performing well
- using time spent waiting
- dropping unwanted tasks
- using unavoidable delays to good advantage.

Further reading and useful websites

Burns R. Unwind. 10 Ways to Manage Stress and Improve your Well-being, 2nd edn. London: Allen & Unwin, 2003.

http://www.time-management-skills-online.com.

Chapter 9

Stress avoidance

Carole Brennan

Aim

The aim of this chapter is to help in identifying and coping with stress, primarily in the workplace.

Outcome

After reading this chapter, readers should have a better understanding of how stress can affect general health and well-being, as well as performance at work. Readers should also have more awareness of the actions that can be taken to develop or adopt appropriate coping strategies.

What is stress?

Stress is different things to different people: to the Olympic athlete, it is the challenge of competing and pushing physical abilities to the limit; to the student, it can be the pressure of examinations; to the leader of the dental team, it may be running the practice; and to the employee, it can be dealing with the boss who is never satisfied. Alternatively, stress may be considered to be the 'wear and tear' our bodies experience as we adjust to our continually changing environment and cope with the many, varied demands of modern society.

We tend to consider stress as harmful, but some stress is good for you, possibly even necessary. While some stress may be good, too much can be detrimental. Too much negative stress results in distress. Negative stress is the stress of losing, failing, overworking, being criticised or generally not coping.

Unfortunately, we all experience negative stress from time to time, and if an individual becomes too stressed their performance suffers. It is impossible to avoid all stress. The only stress-free state is death! The key is to learn how to position yourself at or around the optimal point on the performance–stress graph (Fig 9-1), so that you are coping and performing well and avoiding being stressed to the extent that you are not able to meet aims and objectives, let alone risk suffering a breakdown.

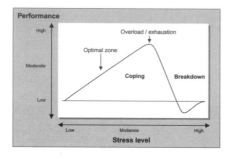

Fig 9-1 Illustration of relationship between performance and level of stress

The optimal point on the performance–stress graph varies from individual to individual, and for any one individual from time to time. Some individuals thrive on high-performance/high-stress working, while others have a much lower performance and stress-related capacity. Under certain conditions, some individuals may suffer an exaggerated reaction, showing disproportionate levels of stress, even at low levels of performance.

Stress at work

Most people have to work and, as a consequence will experience some work-related stress. Some are lucky enough to work in jobs of their choosing and that they enjoy, but others have to work in jobs and in conditions which are not of their choosing and with little, if any, job satisfaction. Whichever situation, there will be periods when an individual may be unhappy, or at least unsettled at work and stressed.

Work-related stress is a major health concern around the world: across all sectors and in all sizes of enterprises. Stress-related breakdown and suicide rates amongst dental healthcare professionals, in particular dental practitioners, are high compared with some other professions, with stress overload being identified as a major contributing factor.

It makes good sense, therefore, to be able to understand what stresses you personally are working under, to be able to recognise when you are distressed and, most importantly, to understand what actions you can take to reduce or control your stress levels.

Understanding stress and its affects

Understanding the process of stress and how it affects you makes it easier to identify your major sources of stress, to know which feelings and reactions indicate your response to stress, and to enable you to anticipate and plan for stressful events or periods.

It does not always follow that moderate to high levels of stress will compromise performance and that stressed people will succumb to physical and psychological ill-health. Stress, however, has been associated with a number of conditions, including high blood pressure, stroke, ulcers, coronary heart disease, asthma, diabetes, cancer and psychiatric disorders such as depression and anxiety (panic) states.

Performance–stress homeostasis describes a state of balance in which the body function efficiently and comfortably. Enhanced stress disturbs this homeostasis by creating an imbalance. It is the ability to cope with stressors that determines the amount of stress that is experienced, and the method of coping with stress that determines whether this stress is damaging (Figs 9-2 and 9-3).

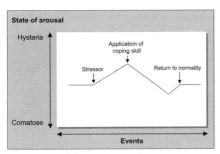

Fig 9-2 Healthy stress reaction.

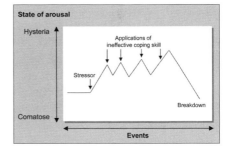

Fig 9-3 Atypical stress reaction.

Most active people prefer to live with a moderate level of arousal and associated stress. Under normal circumstances, a stressor will increase the level of arousal and stress. Sensing this change, the normal reaction is the application of an appropriate coping skill, which may be effective to the extent that it causes the level of arousal and stress to drop below the normal level prior to returning to normal (Fig 9-3). Alternatively, a stressor may trigger an ineffective coping skill or skills, causing the level of arousal and associated stress to peak above, or repeatedly exceed, normal levels, leading eventually to fatigue and breakdown.

The fight or flight response

The fight or flight response is a physiological reaction that prepares the body to respond to an emergency (Fig 9-4). Our distant ancestors needed such reactions to survive the dangers of everyday living. In present circumstances, the fight for flight reaction is still important, but is not normally a matter of life or death.

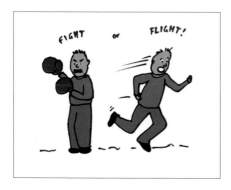

Fig 9-4 The fight or flight response.

This fight or flight response worked perfectly for our ancestors' lifestyle, but today's lifestyle is very different. We live in a fast moving, high-technology world that has evolved considerably faster than we have. Stressors 'threaten us' in every aspect of our lives. Compared with our ancestors, we have to deal with many more stressors and be able to deal with several stressors at the same time. Yet we have only the primitive fight or flight response with which to cope.

Confronted with significant stressors, the body changes, shifting gear into high physiological arousal to enable the fight or flight response to take place. The various processes that take place during the fight or flight response are well documented elsewhere. Following management of the stressor, it takes the body some time to return to the normal state of arousal and associated stress. Reactions that can be associated with this return to normality may include relief, irritability, anxiety, depression or even anger, one or more of which may trigger further stress.

The general adaptation syndrome
If the fight or flight response is constantly being triggered, the body never gets the chance to return to normal and, therefore, remains in a constant state of high arousal with associated stress. This has long-term detrimental effects on our physical and mental health.

Selye, a pioneer in stress research, proposed in 1946 a three-stage process in prolonged stress management, referred to as the general adaptation syndrome. If left untreated, this syndrome predisposes people to various conditions and illnesses.

The sequence runs as follows.

→ *Stage 1: alarm reaction.* Any physical or mental trauma will trigger an immediate set of reactions to stress, such as raised blood pressure and a dry mouth. The immune system is also suppressed and normal levels of resistance are lowered. If the stress is not severe or prolonged, recovery is rapid and, as a consequence, the susceptibility to stress-related conditions is short lived.
→ *Stage 2: resistance.* With repeated exposure to stressors, there is a substantial degree of adaptation. The modified reaction to stress triggers imposes extra demands on the body, which is progressively drained of energy resources and resistance to stress-related disorders and diseases. The individual may become complacent about the high-stress situation, assuming that the body can resist the effects of stress indefinitely. Therein lies the danger: believing in immunity to the effects of stress, and possibly even demanding more of the body, makes an individual increasingly vulnerable to stress-related conditions and illnesses.
→ *Stage 3: exhaustion.* When the body is no longer able to maintain homeostasis and the processes needed to combat stress, there is a sudden fall in the capacity to manage stress, and resistance levels fall. Eventually stress-fighting reserves finally succumb to what Seyle called 'disease adaptation'. In this state, an individual is very vulnerable to stress-related conditions and illnesses.

Signs and symptoms of stress
If some stress is beneficial, how can a person assess if the level of stress they are experiencing is good for them. One of the problems associated with stress is impaired judgement, which blinds us to how well we are controlling and coping with our performance—stress balance. If any of the signs and symptoms

set out in Table 9-1 are being experienced, either continuously or with an increasing frequency, singly or in combination, this may be an indication that you are operating under an unacceptable level of stress.

Table 9-1 **Signs and symptoms of stress**

Physical signs of stress	Behavioural signs of stress
Frequent headaches	Indecisiveness
Indigestion	Forgetting things
Pounding heart	Becoming easily distracted
Breathlessness	Making mistakes
Nausea for no reason	Poor judgement
General lethargy	Quick, ill-judged decision making
Minor aches and pains	Becoming unsociable
Skin rashes	Loss of interest in food, sex, hobbies
Unusual sweating	Insomnia
Constipation or diarrhoea	Aggression

In addition, emotions are a good barometer. If a person reaches the point where very little gives pleasure, and they are constantly nervous, apprehensive and feeling dissatisfied, it is likely that the stress being experiencing is too high or too prolonged.

Managing stress

The goal of stress management is not to eliminate stress, but to determine and control the personal optimum level of stress: creating stress that works for rather than against you.

Determining stress levels and being aware of their effects is not sufficient management. Just as there are many harmful effects of stress, there are many possibilities for its management. All approaches to managing stress require awareness and control, together with changes in attitude and behaviour.

Identifying personal stressors: awareness and reaction

Note your level of stress or distress. Do not ignore it and do not dismiss it. Determine what events stress and distress you, determine what you are saying to yourself about these events (your inner dialogue) and identify how your body responds to different stressors.

Making a stress diary

To fully identify the stressors in your life and your reactions to them, it can be extremely helpful to make a stress diary. As skills and techniques for reducing stress are learnt, the diary can be used to plan the timing of different approaches to stress management.

Each page of the diary is divided into three columns and dated. The columns have the following headings.

- *Stressor.* Activity or event; for example, having to deal with a dispute between members of the dental team.
- *Responses.* What was felt and how the body reacted; for example, 'I felt anxious and tense and could not concentrate on the tasks in hand'.
- *Behaviour.* What was my body language; for example, changes to speech and reaction to those around.

It is important to acknowledge that stressors can be challenging or unpleasant, large or small. Identify whether they arise from external situations or from internal feelings.

It may be useful to add a column to keep track of the place where the stress occurred (home or work) and who or what was involved.

Reviewing the diary should identify emerging patterns.

Identifying personal symptoms of stress

Look at the symptoms set out in Table 9-2, then answer the following questions:

- Do you recognise any of the symptoms as part of your reaction to stressful situations?
- Why do you react in the ways you described in your stress diary? For example, is it easier to be angry and irritable than to take the risk of expressing real feelings?

Table 9-2a **Physical, emotional and intellectual symptoms of stress**

Physical	Emotional	Intellectual
Increased heart rate	Irritability	Forgetfulness
Increased blood pressure	Angry outbursts	Preoccupation
Sweaty palms	Depression	Errors in judging distance
Tightness in chest	Jealousy	Diminished or fantasy
Diarrhoea	Feeling 'uptight'	lifestyle
Tight neck/back muscles	Lowered self-esteem	Reduced creativity
Trembling,	Suspiciousness	Difficulty in making
ticks or twitches	Diminished initiative	decisions
Stuttering	Overalert	Mental confusion
Pupil dilation	Feelings of unreality	Lack of concentration
Nausea and/or vomiting	Loneliness	Diminished productivity
Sleep disturbance	Helplessness	Lack of attention to detail
Fatigue	Insecurity	Orientation to detail
Prone to accidents	Frustration	Oversensitive to criticism
Slumped posture	Lack of interest	
Dryness of mouth	Tendency to cry	
Butterflies in stomach	Reduction of personal	
Susceptibility to minor	involvement	
illnesses	Critical of oneself and	
	others	
	Lack of confidence	
	Self-depreciation	
	Nightmares	
	Exhaustion	
	Tiredness	
	Desire to escape	

Signs of successfully coping with the above symptoms of stress

- ability to carry out tasks efficiently
- ability to take responsibility
- ability to work under authority and rules
- ability to work under difficulties and limitations
- ability to adapt to change
- tolerance of frustration
- reliability

Table 9-2b **Behavioural, health and work symptoms of stress**

Behavioural	Health	Work
Increased smoking	Asthma	Increased absenteeism
Aggressive driving	Coronary heart disease	Increased accident rate
Having accidents	Dizziness	Less job satisfaction
Clumsiness	Headaches/migraine	Poor relationships with
Nervous laughter	Skin complaints	colleagues
Panic	Indigestion	Less commitment to job
Increased alcohol or drug	Aches and pains in chest	Less creativity
use	and limbs	
Carelessness	Diarrhoea	
Eating too much	Frequent urination	
Talking to fast	Nightmares	
Chewing fingernails	Ulcers	
	Loss of sexual interest	

Signs of successfully coping with the above symptoms of stress

- sense of belonging
- ability to show friendliness, respect and love
- ability to take recreation, relax and sleep
- sense of humour
- sense of fulfilment
- sense of self-direction
- reasonable sense of independence and self-reliance
- tolerance of others.

For each sign, think of examples when you experienced these behaviours, feelings or attitudes. Refer to the stress diary, if necessary. Then ask yourself, why do you think some of these coping behaviours or attitudes might be hard to adopt? Examples include that showing friendliness can make you vulnerable to rejection, and that taking on a responsibility makes you responsible for both success and failure.

Taking control of your stress
Once stress reactions and stressors have been identified, it is possible to develop a stress management plan and learn coping strategies.

There are many techniques to help reduce stress, including physical activity, relaxation techniques and indulging in something pleasurable. Such techniques are especially helpful when feeling particularly stressed. In adopting such techniques, it is important to remember that they do not eliminate stressors. Often, people find themselves in situations that are not of their own making. These situations can be potent stressors, particularly if an individual is irritated by or dislikes being in difficult situations. Coping with the stress associated with such situations is strongly linked to self-control.

Beliefs and stress
Consider a situation where you are on your way to work and get caught up in traffic. The delays are so bad that you are going to be very late arriving. By the time you get to work, you are feeling seriously stressed, unprepared and flustered, and for most of the morning you do not perform well.

Responding in this way may stem from a belief that it is unprofessional to be late for work, and that people will be critical of your professionalism. In reality, there is no lack of professionalism, assuming you set off to work in what could be considered to be reasonable time. Professionalism is unquestionably important, but personal views as to what constitutes professional and unprofessional behaviour may need to be changed to limit unnecessary stress.

Some beliefs that may lead to stress are given in Table 9-3. These kinds of belief are defined as barrier beliefs. It is important to identify any barrier beliefs you hold, and to consider changing them to limit unnecessary levels of stress and stressors.

Table 9-3 **The effect of beliefs on stress**

Barrier beliefs: leading to stress	Constructive beliefs: reducing stress
I must cope with everything	I can cope with everything given a reasonable amount of time
Asking for help is a sign of personal weaknesses or failure	I do not have to be able to do everything
Other people's priorities, except those of patients, are more important than mine	My priorities are as important as others
I must keep others happy	Other people are responsible for their feelings; I am responsible for dealing with them fairly and with sensitivity
Telling the truth will lead to upset	I can tell the truth in constructive and productive ways
I have to get things exactly right all the time	I am human; I get things right most of the time and I learn from my mistakes
Work priorities come before all other things	I can balance work with the other things in life which are important to me

So in the situation of heavy traffic, running late and feeling stressed because lateness is a sign of unprofessionalism, it would be much more helpful and realistic to hold the belief that it is important to arrive on time, but professionalism is unaffected by a one-off occurrence caused by factors outwith your control. Needless to say, you apologise to colleagues and patients or clients as and when you arrive at work and take opportunity to explain your lateness. Such openness and honesty should help to relieve the stress you have failed to manage, freeing you up to be efficient and effective the rest of the day.

Consider what beliefs you hold about yourself and work. If any of them are barrier beliefs, then work at changing them. Examples of beliefs that should replace the barrier beliefs are also given in Table 9-3.

Faulty thinking (inner dialogues) and stress
Our beliefs influence the way we think about situations. As a consequence, it is important to identify any faulty thinking processes and to consider how these processes increase stress.

Consider this scenario. You have been putting off telling a colleague that they are being ineffective in dealing with some matter and, in addition, have compounded matters by making a mistake. Having failed to tackle the situation when it first came to light, you are increasing dreading what has to be done, in the knowledge that there will be an angry reaction. Your colleague has a reputation for reacting badly to criticism. As a result, you feel anxious and reluctant to hold the necessary conversation. You avoid the issue for as long as possible, but all the while you are getting more and more stressed.

Alternatively, you could think, 'I don't want to do this, but I may as well get it over and done with and, while I am at it, I may as well raise other issues which I have been putting off tackling'. Now you are feeling angry and resentful so you storm into the situation in a way guaranteed to upset the other person: again, leaving you feeling stressed and unhappy with the outcome.

A much healthy inner dialogue would be, 'I know the reaction will be negative, but I should be able to broach the matter in such a way that it will be viewed as helpful constructive criticism'. This type of inner dialogue is much more likely to result in you speaking to your colleague in a more matter of fact way, sticking to the facts and being firm but fair. Your emotions will be controllable and you avoid getting unnecessarily stressed.

Every time you are faced with a potentially stressful situation, you have a choice: whether to let your thinking run unchecked, and build up the emotions associated with stress, or whether you intervene in that thinking and start to generate positive feelings that will minimise the stress you may experience.

Learn to communicate assertively
Not being able to express your thoughts and feelings in a constructive way often leads to the build up of negative stress. Some people are naturally assertive, while others are more passive, submissive or aggressive. Being passive, submissive or aggressive does nothing to reduce harmful stress levels. Managing such behaviours are dealt with elsewhere in this book (Chapter 10).

Maintain good health
It is generally accepted that high levels of stress may interfere with a person maintaining a healthy lifestyle. Lifestyle characteristics known to increase life expectancy, by 7–10 years in women and 12–15 years in men, can be disrupted by high levels of stress. These characteristics include:

• not smoking
• moderating alcohol consumption
• sleeping around seven hours each day
• eating regular meals with no snacks between meals
• eating at least five portions of fruit and vegetables every day.
• exercising regularly.
• maintaining the recommended body weight.

If levels of stress are driving you to abandon important lifestyle characteristics and, as a consequence, potentially limiting your life expectancy, it is time to take stress management seriously.

Learn to relax
The ability to relax has immediate and long-term benefits. In the short term, relaxation increases the ability to manage stress and enhances feelings of well-being. In the longer term, the ability to relax makes important contributions to quality of life and possibly longevity.

Some people try to relax and relieve feelings of stress by smoking, drinking alcohol, relying on medication or overeating. While these remedies may make some individuals feel better temporarily, they do not remove recurrent stressors. Such activities do not change our personal perceptions, and they do not limit the incidence of stressful events.

When the body responds to relaxation, the effects are opposite to those induced by stress (Fig 9-5).

The ability to relax can be acquired and applied in everyday life. It involves no drugs and can be free of cost. Methods of relaxation vary from individual to individual and can take many forms. The effect is more important than the technique used to achieve the desired outcome.

Develop an effective support system
Another positive behaviour that helps in managing stress is establishing and using an effective support network. Everyone handles stress more effectively

111

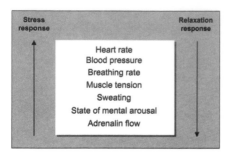

Fig 9-5 The relationship between stress and relaxation responses

if they have other people around, particularly family, friends or other trusted people. The individuals who make excellent supporters include those:

• who are prepared to spend time with you
• who are discreet
• who give frank, honest answers to direct questions
• who are good listeners, with insight and understanding
• who encourage you to be optimistic and hopeful
• who take you seriously and express general concern about your problems.

Improve self-esteem
An important approach to stress management is the ability to be ever hopeful and to see life as a challenge to enjoy. If you are inclined to view yourself negatively and to be self-demeaning, then developing positive attitudes to counteract, if not conquer, harmful stress is all the more difficult.

> In coping with stress, it is important that you develop positive feelings about yourself.

Conclusions

Stress is the wear and tear our bodies experience as we adjust to our continually changing environment. Some stress is necessary to perform well in everyday lives. There are many causes of stress in today's society, just as there are many signs and symptoms of stress.

A key step in managing stress is identifying your stressors. It is possible to reduce and manage stress by various activities, developing and adopting a variety of stress management strategies and, above all else, raising confidence and self-esteem.

Reference

Selye H. The general adaptation syndrome and the diseases of adaptation. J Clin Endocrinol 1946;6:117–231.

Further reading and useful websites

Back K, Back K. Assertiveness at Work, 3rd edn. Maidenhead, UK: McGraw-Hill, 1999.

Burns R. Unwind. 10 Ways to Manage Stress and Improve your Well-being, 2nd edn. London: Allen & Unwin, 2003.

Chapter 10
Handling disputes

Carole Brennan and Marina Harris

Aim

The aim of this chapter is to consider how to remain assertive in the face of aggressive and non-assertive behaviour from other people in the workplace.

Outcome

The chapter should lead to an understanding of the role that aggressive and non-assertive behaviour plays in influencing interpersonal relationships. Readers should be able to identify the features of aggressive behaviour and the various negative effects of non-assertive behaviour and be able to formulate assertive responses to counteract aggression and non-assertive behaviour.

Introduction

Assertive behaviour can help in making an individual a happy, effective team member. It must be recognised, however, that assertiveness can, on occasions, be a risk when other people behave aggressively or non-assertively. This chapter concentrates on how to remain assertive when others are trying to adversely influence your behaviour.

Aggressive behaviour

Most people find it difficult or uncomfortable being the subject of aggression from others. Responding to aggression in a way that defuses the situation, and hopefully goes at least some way to resolving the cause, is an important skill (Fig 10-1).

Levels of aggression

There are two levels of aggression that can be clearly identified.

- *Higher-level aggression.* This usually takes the form of personal attacks; for example, 'That's just typical of you' or 'That's not true and well you know

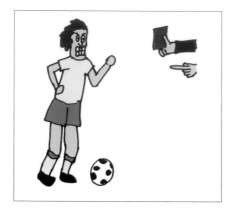

Fig 10-1 Aggression in behaviour.

it'. People who use this form of aggressive behaviour are being aggressive towards the person and not the issue.

- *Lower-level aggression.* Lower level aggression can take the form of sarcasm, accusations, being dismissive of a person or a statement, or by being patronising, not listening, or dominating a conversation.

Handling aggressive behaviour

The aim of handling colleague's aggression is to deal with the issues and feel positive about the interaction afterwards. Outlined below are steps to be taken in standing your ground in the face of aggression. The main aim is to defuse the aggression in the aggressor.

Step one

The first step is critical. Mustering and maintaining resolve at this stage increases considerably the chances of responding assertively. Taking a few, slow deep breaths buys you critical seconds to gather yourself and your thoughts for your response. In addition, a few more seconds of thought can be achieved by using starters such as 'Yes', 'Well, OK' or 'I appreciate you have a problem'. Slowing everything down from the outset greatly reduces the risk of your initial response triggering even more aggression from the aggressor.

Step two

When people are being aggressive towards you, it is possible that they take you by surprise. Their words tend to come out very quickly and may not even be coherent. Following the initial tirade, begin to respond by asking questions in an assertive manner. To do this, keep your voice firm, clear and evenly paced. Slowing your response down may even encourage the other person to slow down, diffusing their anger, allowing you to begin to understand the issue. Start asking questions. This usually has an effect on the aggressor, as they will have to listen to your questions and think of answers. Slowing things down creates thinking time for both parties, with the possibility of the aggressor toning down the attack.

Sometimes, the aggressor may be so pent up that you are unable to get a word in edgeways. If this is the case, do not interrupt, let the aggressor get the matter off their chest; eventually they will run out of steam. Once this has happened, the exchange has a better chance of becoming an 'assertive–assertive one'.

Some questions that you may consider asking include:

- When did this happen?
- Why do you say that?
- Why do you think this happened?
- Can you give me some specific examples?
- What actually happened?

If at this stage, the aggressor remains aggressive, with little if any let up, encourage a full airing of the grievance before moving on to step three:

Step three
At the third stage, you should begin to say more about where you stand on the issue, while at the same time showing that you understand the other person's position. The aggressor may well begin to feel that they are getting through to you, even though you have indicated that your position differs from theirs. This will not necessarily stop the aggressor from trying to influence you, but at least it will be done in a less heated manner. If this happens, the aggressor's behaviour should become less aggressive and more assertive. Ways of stating your standpoint assertively could be to make the following types of statement:

- I don't believe that I have ignored you, but I'd like to hear why you feel I have
- I can see that you have strong feelings about this; however, I do see it differently, given that…

The responsive behaviours in steps two and three form a powerful combination. Faced with such assertion, it is often difficult for people to

117

continue to be aggressive. If, however, the person continues to be aggressive, you move on to step four.

Step four
If the aggressor persists with, or reverts to their aggression, then it is time to step up your assertion. Here you put the emphasis on your position.

The first option may simply be to repeat your earlier assertive statement in respect of your position, or you may wish to change your statement in light of the new information you have gained as a result of asking questions. To give strength to the restatement of your position, slow it down and lay emphasis on the key words, especially if you feel that the aggressor has ignored you earlier.

An alternative at this stage is to point out that past agreements, stemming from aggressive behaviour, have been broken, or that the other person's behaviour is unacceptable. For example, it may be appropriate to say:

- I see it differently,
- On the one hand you say you want to improve relationships within the team, but on the other hand you are saying the team cannot work. Now, let's look afresh at the problem.

Step five
If you have worked at being assertive, with no change in the aggressor's aggressive behaviour, you may begin to experience strong feelings of frustration, resentment or annoyance. These strong emotions can be a barrier to your own assertiveness and may lead to you becoming aggressive or non-assertive. It is, therefore, important to appreciate when to express your feelings to the aggressor.

Alternatively, you may feel it important to state the consequence of the continued aggressive behaviour, by saying, for example:

- If you continue to shout in this way, I will put the phone down and call you back
- If you continue to be aggressive and threatening, I will have no choice but to ask you to leave.

At this stage, the other person will hopefully see that you mean business.

Step six
If all your efforts have been to no avail, you may be thinking, 'Well that's it, I've tried everything else, now, I can become aggressive without feeling guilty'. You still, however, have two options open to you. The first option is to cut off the interaction. You may already have warned the aggressor of this in the previous step. A simple statement such as, 'I don't feel we are making any progress. Let's meet again soon, when we have both had time to reflect', may be sufficient.

Cutting off the interaction alerts the other person to the effect of their behaviour on you. Also, it makes it clear to them that you are not prepared to take their sustained aggression.

The second option is to put the immediate matter aside and to look at the underlying issue or feelings that are causing the aggression. This may be achieved by saying:

• 'We need to stop and consider what is causing this difficulty.'

A useful rule of thumb is to move up a step only if the aggression continues. Aggression can usually be diffused early in the stepped process. Knowing that you have further options available to you can increase your confidence to behave with firmer assertiveness.

Non-assertive behaviour

We are quick to recognise people using aggressive behaviour towards us, but typically relatively slow to appreciate the use of non-assertive behaviour to influence us. Non-assertive behaviour is less dramatic and apparent than aggression, but equally damaging.

When people are behaving non-assertively, it can be frustrating, causing you to behave in a non-assertive or even aggressive manner. Such a response will have a negative impact on the outcome of the situation.

Effects of non-assertive behaviour
On the individual
When people behave non-assertively they are aiming to avoid conflict and to please everyone. Their behaviour may, however, have the opposite effect. An individual who frequently behaves in a non-assertive manner suffers from a growing loss of self-esteem, with increasing inability to deal with situations

let alone take initiatives. In time, they begin to feel angry, frustrated, hurt or self-pitying. These feelings are directed inwards, causing the individual to become stressed and susceptible to psychosomatic problems such as head-aches or backaches.

On others

Initially, people tend to feel sorry for individuals who behave non-assertively. They may begin to feel guilty about asking the non-assertive person to do things, knowing that they will agree but then fail to cope. After a while, people start to feel irritated by sustained non-assertion. The behaviour may, however, have an effect opposite to that intended and lead to doubts about the integrity of the person. It is a paradox that the person who sets out to please often ends up being less respected than an aggressive person.

> A person setting out to please often becomes less respected than an aggressive person.

On the workplace

Some of the following situations caused by non-assertive behaviour in the workplace may be familiar:

- conflicts and disputes are not managed successfully, leaving members of the team feeling disgruntled and angry
- difficult decisions may be avoided or delayed, causing the team to miss deadlines and be inefficient and possibly ineffective
- few initiatives are taken, the team does not keep up to date and opportunities are lost, resulting in loss of business and demotivated staff.

Sooner or later, the leader of the team will over-react, possibly with aggression, to re-establish authority, often choosing the wrong issue on which to take a stand. Such situations may spiral out of control.

Different forms of non-assertive behaviour

Non-assertive behaviour takes different forms:

Silent non-assertion

Individuals who use silent non-assertion fail to raise important issues, to state a disagreement or to express their feelings and wishes. This form of non-assertion is difficult to detect (Fig 10-2). Indications of this behaviour include:

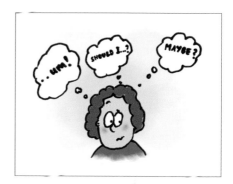

Fig 10-2 Non-assertive behaviour.

- lack of eye contact
- doubtful facial expressions
- shuffling body movements and restlessness.

Tentativeness
Tentativeness is indicated by reactions such as, 'Oh I suppose so', 'Maybe your right' or 'Well, it might be OK'. Anything to avoid conflict and usually intended to please.

Doubting
Comments such as 'I'm not really sure about that' or 'That may be a bit awkward' reflect the doubter who wishes to play safe and test your reaction. If challenged, the doubter will retract. If encouraged, they may reluctantly express a view.

Avoidance
The avoider tends to respond to requests with excuses such as 'I haven't really got time' or 'I would, only I'm rushed off my feet'. Time and overwork are the more common smokescreens to hide lack of confidence or ability. In the case of such individuals, non-assertive behaviour needs to be distinguished from laziness.

Indecision
Statements such as 'Oh, I don't really mind' or 'Whatever suits you best' reflects the indecisive person unwilling to take responsibility. They often do have a preference but are unwilling to state it, and they may complain if you make a decision they dislike.

Complaining
Complaining can be about you, 'Oh no, not another job to do'. Such complaints may be made directly to you or within earshot, with the aim of making you feel guilty. Complaints can also be made to you about a third party, where the complainant is trying to enlist your support. As they are often unwilling to take any action themselves, they prefer to encourage others to do their complaining for them.

Uncertainty
Comments such as 'I thought I might' or 'Do you think I should?' indicate a person unwilling to make a decision based on judgement. Uncertain, non-assertive behaviour is indicative of lack of self-confidence.

Helplessness and self-pity
Expressions such as 'What's the use of?' or 'I'll never get this sorted out' are aimed at making you feel sorry for individuals. Such individuals see themselves as powerless to change, let alone influence their working environment.

Self put-downs
Self put-downs may be used because there is a genuine lack of confidence or ability: 'I'm hopeless at this', 'You know me', 'I'm bound to get it all wrong'. More often than not, these are expressed as exaggerations or to understate capabilities in an effort to avoid doing something or to avoid criticism.

Sacrificing
Being over-helpful by offering to work through lunch, stay late or to take work home may be indicative of self-sacrificing non-assertiveness. The individual is trying to please you, sometimes trying to put you in their debt so you will feel grateful, or sometimes wanting to make you feel guilty knowing that they are going out of their way for you, ignoring their own needs and wishes.

Handling non-assertive behaviour
Managing non-assertive behaviour includes respecting the rights, needs, wants and opinions of others. This means getting to know and understand the individual's needs, wants and opinions. This is sometimes difficult when the person is being non-assertive. The aim in managing non-assertive behaviour is to encourage the individual to behave more positive. Some assertive responses and comments that may help in coping with someone indulging in non-assertive behaviour are set out in Table 10-1.

122

Table 10-1 **Examples of assertive responses to non-assertive behaviour**

Non-assertive behaviour	Assertive response	Comments
Tentative agreement	You seem to be hesitating, what's the difficulty?	You need to find out if there is a problem and what it is before you can get a firm commitment
Tentatively expressing doubts: 'That... er... may leave me with a bit of a problem'	What is the problem? Lets see if we can sort it out	This makes it clear that you realise there may be a genuine problem but that it need not get in the way
Stating excuses: 'Well, I don't seem to be able to find the time to get started on it'	Oh, I see. Well, I think there may be a way around that. Is there any other problem?'	Sometimes it is difficult to distinguish an excuse from a real reason. This response avoids using words like 'Oh that's just an excuse' or 'What is the real reason?' These may make the other person think you are accusing them of lying
Proposals at own expense: 'I suppose I can do the work during lunch/at home/over the weekend'	I'm glad you mentioned your workload. Can we look for ways to reduce this so that you don't have to work during lunch/at home/over the weekend?	This enables you to avoid feeling guilty, sorry, or overgrateful for making what is a reasonable request
Putting self down: 'I'm hopeless at this, I made a real mess of it last time'	I don't agree that you are hopeless at this. The last time was not good, but I believe you can do it well. What specific problems did you have with it?	Important to counter exaggerations with a more realistic assessment – no effusive praise. Then give assurance to improve confidence – avoid 'pep' talks ('You'll be alright' or 'Don't worry') as treating like a child only encourages more non-assertive behaviour
Enhancing others at own expense: 'You're very good at that; I seem to find it difficult and time consuming'	What makes it so difficult and time consuming for you?	This avoids the negative comparisons and looks at the facts

When dealing with aggression, it is usually possible to modify the aggressive behaviour to an assertive level. When dealing with non-assertive behaviour, however, it is sometimes unrealistic to get the person to behave assertively.

The use of feedback techniques to manage behaviour

Feedback is information on performance. The technique of feedback has two very useful characteristics:

- it feeds information both ways between two people
- it works especially well for resolving behavioural and personality difficulties.

Learning to use feedback techniques facilitates dealing with various issues in the workplace environment.

Why feedback?

What has feedback got that other techniques lack? The major advantage of feedback is that it is a two-way, non-confrontational technique. The technique is designed to be able to tackle difficult topics in a positive way, without either party feeling the need to be aggressive or defensive. In addition it:

- has a high success rate
- tends to encourage a full and frank exchange of views and concerns
- engenders confidence and team working.

Planning a feedback meeting

As a feedback session is intended to be at most semi-formal, non-confrontational and ideally open ended, it should be at a time when the discussion will not be rushed and there is opportunity to complete the process with agreed actions.

Further arrangements include:

- choosing a place where there will be no interruption and, if necessary, put a 'Do not disturb' sign on the closed door and arrange for telephone calls to be diverted; an enclosed office or meeting room is preferred
- turn off computers, mobile phones and other electronic devices to avoid distractions
- arrange refreshments and ensure that the room is comfortable in terms of seating and temperature.

Preparation
Before the meeting takes place, think carefully through and list the key points you wish to make, and how you are going to word them in a non-confrontational and constructive way. Thoughtless wording of remarks may make the meeting confrontational and, as a consequence, detract from the outcome.

The person you are meeting with may, quite reasonably, want some examples of the kind of behaviour to be discussed. Identify these ahead of the meeting.

Making the most of the meeting
It is best to start the meeting with some informalities to settle into the meeting and the environment. In the process of this preamble, it is important for both parties to agree that they wish the meeting to be constructive. If there is animosity, let alone aggression from the outset, it is usually best to recognise that the session should be rescheduled. If there is mutual agreement to proceed with the meeting, be prepared to listen and to reflect before answering questions. If there is lack of clarity or understanding, go back and clarify matters as you go along. Record only the agreed outcomes and actions and any specific points on which there is mutual agreement to note for future reference. If the meeting becomes prolonged, or if any of the topics raised cause an adverse reaction, take a break for 10 to 15 minutes and reconvene. During the discussion, remain focused and remember to express yourself in a non-confrontational way, otherwise the meeting will, in all probability, fail to achieve its purpose. The following points may help to facilitate a positive outcome.

→ *Avoid provocative expressions.* Use of such comments such as 'You irritate people,' or 'You don't seem to care' is likely to trigger a response of denial. There is then a stand-off situation, which will detract from the usefulness of the meeting.
→ *Do not exaggerate.* You lose credibility if you say 'You always...' or 'You never...'. The use of inappropriate superlatives, such as huge, devastating, unimaginable or unforgivable, is also likely to create a negative response. If you say and mean such things, the opportunity for any workable resolution is very limited.
→ *Avoid being judgemental.* It may be very tempting and satisfying, but it is not useful.
→ *Do not label.* Making remarks such as 'You are negative' or 'You are ineffective' is not helpful. To avoid making these kinds of statement, focus on the person's behaviour, rather than their personality.

→ *Take time.* Do not be rushed; take time to think and to choose your words. It is far better to take time than to hurriedly say something which may offend or deserve an unhelpful response.

Identifying solutions
The feedback session is about agreeing a way forward through a series of solutions, rather than identifying more problems. Possible solutions should be suggested, discussed and refined before being agreed. Some suggested solutions may be best 'slept on' and revisited; others may be immediately acceptable. In discussing and agreeing solutions, both parties must keep an open mind; closed thinking is unlikely to move matters on.

Concluding the meeting
Following a recap and noting the agreed solutions and actions, it is important to discuss a follow-up meeting and its timing. Finally, it is good to conclude a feedback session by reflecting on how well the meeting has gone and how it could be improved on the next occasions.

Conclusions

Aggression and non-assertive behaviour are regrettably common occurrences in the workplace. If left unchecked, both behaviours sooner or later lead to disputes, compromising the efficiency and effectiveness of the team effort. Careful management of aggression and non-assertive behaviour using techniques such as feedback techniques is important to the future cohesion and working of the workplace team. Feedback sessions should focus on resolutions rather than identifying more problems, let alone aggravating existing tensions. Above all else, disputes are better prevented rather than being dealt with, as and when they arise. A proactive rather than a reactive approach is a simpler method to preserve and hopefully strengthen team unity and performance.

Further reading

Back K, Back K. Assertiveness at Work, 3rd edn. Maidenhead, UK: McGraw-Hill, 1999.

Burns R. Unwind. 10 Ways to Manage Stress and Improve your Well-being, 2nd edn. London: Allen & Unwin, 2003.

Jay R. How To Manage Your Boss. London: Prentice Hall Business, 2002.

Chapter 11

Companies and commerce

Gail Vernon

Aim

The aim of this chapter is to outline the benefits of working collaboratively with the dental trade to benefit both the dental team and patients.

Outcome

The chapter should increase awareness of the benefits to the dental practice of working with the dental trade in a collaborative manner.

Introduction

Dentistry is increasingly 'big business'. Dental practices and dental laboratories spend large amounts of money on products, materials and equipment, purchasing from a large number of dental companies, including manufactures, distributors and service providers, collectively called the 'dental trade'.

Assuming that a dental professional is looking for better ways to promote oral health and learn about modern approaches to oral healthcare provision, this will be assisted by identifying and then selecting suppliers from a wide range of manufacturers, wholesalers and distributors. The dental industry serves the needs of the entire dental care team, supporting them in a number of ways to deliver a high quality service and safe, effective care for their patients.

Choosing a company to do business with

There are literally thousands of companies across the world that supply products and services to dentistry. Increasingly, dental practices and laboratories are targeted with product and service information by telephone, direct mail, through the dental press or by visiting sales representatives. With so many companies demanding time, how does a dental team decided which ones they would like to do business with, and in what ways?

Dental trade associations
Most countries have a dental trade association. These associations are the bodies that represent manufacturers, wholesalers and distributors who market products and services to the dental industry. By way of example of what to expect from a trade association member and to outline the benefits of dealing with companies that are trade association members, the British Dental Trade Association (BDTA) will be considered.

The BDTA, representing the UK dental industry, provides members with a range of services and benefits designed to enhance the performance of the industry, and dentistry in general. The BDTA relationship to dental care providers within the UK is summarised in the following statement: 'To provide the best service to your patients, you need dependable support from your suppliers. BDTA members fulfil this need for the whole dental team.'

This is achieved by a set of commitments.

→ *Commitment to quality.* Member companies must adhere to an agreed code of practice. This is an indication that member companies are actively engaged in creating and maintaining industry standards.
→ *Commitment to training.* Member companies are encouraged to participate in professional training initiatives. The Dental Industry Training Institute (DITI) is the training arm of the BDTA. Under the BDTA's Code of Practice, members are responsible for ensuring that their staff are appropriately trained and have the experience, product knowledge and ability necessary to perform their duties properly and effectively. These duties include, for example, effective and timely responses to customer enquiries.
→ *Commitment to service.* The BDTA acts as a conciliatory body for dental professionals if high standards are not being maintained, or in the event of a dispute.

Benefits of working with companies
Many companies within the dental industry offer a range of resources and benefits to the dental team. If the company can interact and, therefore, get closer to the customer, they can better understand the customer's requirements. This will give the company the opportunity to propose products and services that are relevant to the professional's role or field of dentistry, and thereby work with customers to mutual advantage and the benefit of patients. By working collaboratively with chosen dental

companies, the professional can receive a range of added-value benefits that can help in more fully meeting the expectations of patients.

Interactions with companies

Visits from company representatives
Company representatives, as discussed in more detail in Chapter 12, can offer a number of useful services. In particular, experienced representatives who are specialists in their field can supply a wealth of information. They may visit on a regular basis to leave product samples, quickly and efficiently update the dental team on the latest products or services offered by their company, provide product training in respect of both new and existing materials and equipment, and contribute to the induction and initial instruction of new members of the dental care team. Time spent with company representatives may prove valuable for continuing professional development, albeit of a general rather than verifiable nature. Given that company representatives travel between practices and laboratories, they may be able to assist in issues such as looking for a new member of staff, obtaining third party references and understanding how colleagues have best used products or services. Knowing how to get the most out of visits by company representatives and making representatives feel valued is an important dental team skill.

Lunch and learn events
Many companies offer 'lunch and learn' events. These events provide an opportunity for the dental team to learn about products and services offered by a company. A major advantage of this approach to relating to company representatives is the opportunity to minimise loss of chairside time. The real benefit, however, is that the team can take time to listen to a presentation together and ask questions as a group. Furthermore, the session can be tailored to meet particular interests and requirements. The company may also provide refreshments, typically in the form of a sandwich or similar form of lunch.

Loyalty schemes
Loyalty schemes exist to reward customers for repeat business. Schemes may offer points that can be collected against purchases and redeemed for products, discounts or gifts. Loyalty schemes allow manufactures and suppliers to monitor your buying habits. This information can help to tailor a dental trade service to best suit your ongoing needs.

Exhibition support

Companies are frequently approached to provide support at trade shows, training events and various dental meetings (Fig 11-1). From the company's point of view, it is beneficial to have opportunity to see a number of existing and possible new customers together at one venue, and to be seen to be supporting training, lifelong learning and related activities, let alone the profession in general. It is important, however, that members of the dental team attending supported events take time to visit the trade show and interact with the trade. In this way, the trade gets value for money and will be encouraged to continue to support such events.

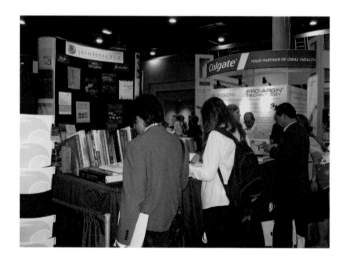

Fig 11-1 A trade show.

Advertising

There are an increasing number of dental publications, ranging from magazines circulated free of charge to the dental team to subscription journals, many of which are linked to membership of a national or international professional organisation, including specialist societies.

Many companies advertise their products and services in a range of dental publications. The revenue from this advertising contributes to production, printing and distribution costs. In return, companies are seeking opportunities to update members of the dental team on their range of products and services. Many publications include a reader's response scheme, which allows readers to request further information and samples of products and services advertised. This gives feedback to the companies, including reassurance that they are reaching their intended audience. Such feedback may also be obtained by requesting details of where clients learnt about products and services when placing orders.

Marketing to patients

Patients are consumers and as such are exposed to a huge amount of information. They may be influenced by a wide range of advertising and educational material in everyday life. Patients are increasingly aware of the benefits of good oral health and the advancements in available treatments. This, together with increasing awareness of dental attractiveness, means that patients have probably never been more motivated to understand modern dental care and to seek more advanced forms of treatment. Many companies develop marketing materials that help to increase the usage of their products or services. These materials include waiting room posters and patient information leaflets designed specifically to help practices to increase the awareness of treatments and products which may be of interest to patients. Some companies and organisations have national and international events and campaigns to promote good oral health. Initiatives in the UK such as 'Smile Week' and 'Oral Health Month' promote oral health and its many advantages and are supported by joint working between the dental trade and the professional.

New products

Dental companies make large investments in the research and development of new products and services. These investments are intended to boost sales, enhance the delivery of care to patients, or to combat dental disease and thereby change treatment needs. An example of ongoing investment is the development of products to be used by the patient at home, particularly oral hygiene aids developed for preventive treatments. Clinical trials to show the effectiveness of new products, an important element of new product research and development, are largely financed by manufacturers. Findings from these trials directly or indirectly benefit many millions of people around the world, with spin-off benefits of new understanding and knowledge of dental diseases and their management. In today's cost-sensitive market, however, many generic products have been introduced that undercut the price of branded products. While there may be short-term, cost-containing gains to be made through the purchase of generic products, reduced returns to manufacturers endanger professional support programmes, limit the investment in new research and development and, in turn, contain product and service enhancement. In other words, a profitable dental market is one in which manufacturer, supplier and consumer have the opportunity to work together to great effect, ultimately in the interests of patients. Collaborative working, mutual understanding and shared goals may, therefore, be considered to be key elements of the relationship between the profession and dental trade. Such working is critical to meeting the ever-increasing challenge of modern oral healthcare provision.

Further reading and useful websites

British Dental Trade Association www.bdta.org.uk/.

Chapter 12
Working with company representatives
Gail Vernon

Aim

This chapter discusses how to select which representatives to take time to see and how to build collaborative relationships with key contacts; this has many benefits, including continuous quality improvement, good clinical outcomes and enhanced patient satisfaction.

Outcome

This chapter will assist members of the dental team to become familiar with ways in which to assess the merits of different company representatives, and ways in which to work with selected representatives to best possible advantage.

Introduction

As the dental market continues to grow in value and size, there are an ever-increasing number of company representatives calling on dental practices and laboratories. These company representatives offer a wide and expanding range of services, equipment and products to support the dental team in various ways.

A representative of a company should be fully acquainted with company products and arrangements for conducting business. Some are limited to sales and, as a consequence, should know their products and services in great detail. Others may be more technically orientated, with expertise in demonstrating the use of equipment and materials. An example of this would be a dental technician representative who demonstrates the use of porcelain in the construction of crown and bridgework. An experienced representative should have a wealth of information that is helpful to the entire dental team. As the relationship builds, so does the trust and mutual understanding. The representative then becomes a valuable resource for all members of the dental team.

> Company representatives should have specialist knowledge and understanding in their field of business.

Since time is a precious resource, it is not possible to see every representative that walks through the door, especially if the visit is unscheduled (cold calling). It is best to develop mutually beneficial relationships with representatives of selected companies who you have confidence in and do business with on a regular basis. These relationships should enhance the support that you receive in terms of service and effective use of your time. Most practices have a number of established contacts that visit on a regular basis. Take some time to review each of these contacts critically in terms of the benefits that they bring to the practice or laboratory. Such a review may take the form of a team discussion, with a view to forming a consensus. Alternatively, the team may wish to draw up a check list of types of support and services required, and then check the various elements off against each company and representative. The checklist may include the following:

- Do we receive regular visits?
- Is the representative knowledgeable?
- Does the representative provide new information and added value at each visit?
- Does the company understand and meet the need of the team?
- Does the company get back to the team when additional information is requested?
- Does the representative respect time?
- Do they give good service?
- Do the products and services meet needs and expectations?
- Does the company support reasonable requests for samples?
- Does the company have information resources to share with patients?
- Is the company a member of the national dental trade association?
- Do we get any additional benefits from time taken to see the representative?

Although this list is not exhaustive, it should help to identify under-performing and alternative companies. Looking at each question in turn:

Do we receive regular visits?
Does the representative visit the practice or telephone on a regular basis: monthly, quarterly or when requested? It is human nature to support people that support you; therefore, companies that have representatives who call on a regular basis, rather than at random, may be more appropriate for building

a relationship. At each visit or during a telephone call, the representative should arrange the next contact. Some representatives have stickers to put in diaries or on wall calendars to remind the dental team when they are next in town. This helps to plan meetings more effectively, let alone give opportunity to change the appointment if other commitments create a clash of dates.

Do we have a knowledgeable representative?
Does the representative give good, useful and relevant information about their products and services? Reliable, accessible and easily assimilated information can be invaluable. Representatives and companies capable of providing such information, ideally in different formats, can greatly enhance efficiency and effectiveness in a practice or laboratory. A relationship built on real cost benefits can be most constructive, with many spin-off benefits, including enhanced patient care.

Does the representative provide new information and added value at each visit?
Is there good reason for a visit and a call on your time? It may be that the representative has information on a new product, news in respect of an established product or details of special offers, or it may be that the representative is simply checking that all is well with their client. The dental team should indicate the basis on which a visit will be welcome. If visits to simply check that all is well are unwelcome, or should be replaced by a telephone call, then the representative should be advised accordingly.

Does the representative understand and meet the needs of the team?
Does the representative take the time to learn about the practice and find out what your requirements are, rather than working to their own agenda? Do they ask relevant questions and provide good answers? If so, this is when a representative becomes a resource, rather than just a salesperson.

Does the company get back to the team when additional information is requested?
Depending on many factors, including level of experience and the size of their product range, the representative may not be able to answer every question you pose during a visit. When they say they will get back to you with an answer, do they honour such commitments? A company which honours commitments engenders trust and, in turn, a good working relationship. Failures 'to deliver' are frustrating and time wasting and, as a result, have cost consequences.

Does the representative respect time?
When you agree to take time out of your day to meet a representative, do they respect your time? If you let them know that you have only 10 minutes,

do they keep to that, or run over, leaving you running behind? A good representative recognises that your time is precious, works within time restrictions and gives the client the option to terminate the visit or call. As a consequence, you will be prepared to see them again, rather than finding excuses to avoid future contacts.

Do they give good service?

Following a contact or transaction with a company, the dental team should feel satisfied and well served. There is a saying that 'people buy people'. You may enjoy seeing the representative, but do not have a need or desire to adopt or increase the usage of their product or service. Alternatively, you may wish to use or increase your reliance on a product or service but have reservations given the approach, professionalism, knowledge or attitude of the representative. Answering this question, and acting accordingly, will help the dental team to manage their time more effectively, in particular if alternative suppliers would welcome the business.

Do the products and services meet needs and expectations?

To be able to assess if products and services meet needs and expectations, it may be necessary from time to time to shop or ask around, or to undertake audits and other forms of review. It is all too easy to stay with familiar products and services when, with a small amount of effort, different, better-quality products and services can be identified. Just because a product has served you well for a number of years does not mean that it is the best available.

Does the company support reasonable requests for samples?

If samples are applicable and available, does the representative anticipate and meet your needs or leave you frustrated with, for example, intermittent supplies and the need to ration or be highly selective in the provision of samples to patients? If the latter, samples can become a nuisance rather than a benefit. Equally, if the dental team is swamped with samples, particularly samples it does not want, then nuisance levels may well exceed benefit.

Does the company have information resources to share with the patient?

If a company has a product or service that you wish to promote to patients, are you supported in realising this goal? Support may be in the form of patient samples, information leaflets, posters for the waiting room and good-quality websites. The commitment of a company may be judged from how up to date its resources are.

Is the company a member of the national dental trade association?
The value of the national dental trade association (the British Dental Trade
Association in the UK) is discussed in more detail in Chapter 12.

Further reading and useful websites

British Dental Trade Association www.bdta.org.uk/

Chapter 13
Professionalism
What is professionalism?

Nairn Wilson

Aim

The aim of this chapter is to consider professionalism in dentistry, with special emphasis on the dental team.

Outcomes

This chapter will provide insight into professionalism as it relates to all members of the dental team, with pointers as to how professionalism should be developed to meet the every changing and increasing expectations of society.

Introduction

There is no widely recognised, all-embracing definition of professionalism, let alone a definition specific to dentistry. Furthermore, the concept of professionalism continues to evolve to reflect changes in society in respect of values and expectations. That said, few would contest the following statement: professionalism is fulfilling all the expectations of being a member of a profession, having a vocation or calling that involves expertise or a high level of understanding, practised and typically regulated according to a set of standards, expectations or obligations. The expectations and obligations of being a member of the dental profession vary little from country to country. These expectations and obligations are embodied in the six principles that underpin being a dental professional:

- putting patient's interests first and acting to protect them
- respecting patient's dignity and choices
- protecting the confidentiality of patient's information
- cooperating with other members of the dental team and other healthcare colleagues in the interests of the patient
- maintaining professional knowledge and competence
- being trustworthy.

To add to the above, society in general expects amongst other qualities, a professional person to be:

- respectable: to behave in an appropriate manner
- responsible: to act in reasonable, considered ways
- reliable: to honour commitments and keep promises
- honest: to always tell the truth
- robust in terms of their professional integrity: an unswerving commitment to professionalism.

Quite a list of obligations and expectations, but society looks for such wide-ranging commitment if individuals are to be afforded the privilege of classifying themselves as professionals and to claim membership of a profession.

Professionalism: a way of life

Professionalism is not limited to time spent in the clinical environment; it is a 24/7 commitment. This is not to say that a professional person can never relax and enjoy themselves. When they do, however, it should not be in a way which causes offence or brings the profession into disrepute. Professionalism is, at all time, an individual responsibility of members of the profession and of the profession as a whole. It becomes a way of life that is reflected, first and foremost, in putting patients first and, in a more general context, in being a good citizen with a social conscience.

> Professionalism is a 24/7 commitment.

Professionalism in working life

Professionalism involves many complex relationships. These include relationships with patients, colleagues and other members of the dental team, and with individuals who support and otherwise facilitate the work of the team. The interactions and influences of these relationships are constantly changing with time and circumstances, often on a day-to-day basis. They need to be the subject of checks and balances to keep them in a stable, albeit dynamic, equilibrium. This demands constant awareness of personal behaviours towards others, personal reactions to challenges and threatening situations, and the views others form of you, both as a fellow human being and as a member of the profession. The dentist as the leader of the dental team has special responsibilities in this regard – leadership by example.

The other major aspects of professionalism in personal matters include professionalism in clinical practice, spanning its many varied forms, and professionalism in conducting all relevant business transactions. The maxim in such matters is 'always treat people the way you would wish to be treated'. Success in achieving these goals generates and justifies trust. Any abuse of trust is a major breach of professionalism, with the inevitable negative effects on the standing of the individual and the profession as a whole. Doing the right thing, the right way, at the right time, with the right outcome underpins professionalism in professional matters. This requires well-developed, self-awareness, including being alert to:

• personal and professional strengths and weaknesses
• variations in personal motivation and attitudes
• personal biases and the influence of personal beliefs and cultural background
• personality traits and reactions to different types of people, circumstances and situations.

> Professionalism means always treating people the way you would wish to be treated.

No healthcare professional is perfect, let alone superhuman, and consequently suffers from certain failings and limitations, often occurring as occasional minor lapses in otherwise good, if not exemplary professional behaviour. Recognising when such lapses occur and having the honesty and integrity to admit to them if they do, and to take appropriate remedial action, shows great strength of conviction to professionalism. More often than not, all that is required to demonstrate professionalism in the face of some lapse in behaviour is to be 'big enough' to apologise appropriately. Furthermore, subsequent to the event, there is a need to reflect on what caused the lapse in behaviour and to take steps to prevent a recurrence.

Professionalism to students and new members of the profession may seem to be a demanding, ever-present challenge to temper personal behaviour and act differently from peers in other walks of life – a threat to self-expression and, in many cases, new-found autonomy. This may well be the reality of the situation, but given the opportunities afforded by a career in a healthcare profession, being professional is a small price to pay.

Professionalism in personal life

Professionalism in personal matters spans personal conduct, morality and decency and social responsibility. What is considered to be acceptable and, more importantly, unacceptable in such matters differs from person to person: what may be acceptable and unremarkable to one person may be quite unacceptable and reprehensible to another. By way of a guide, it is important to consider what is acceptable and unacceptable behaviour to the majority of reasonable people. In suggesting such an approach, it is to be remembered that not all people are reasonable and in reality 'there is no pleasing all the people all of the time'; however, this should not stop a professional from trying to achieve this goal. Behaviour often needs to be modified according to circumstances; for example, to take account of cultural sensitivities within different groups of people. In today's multicultural society, this requires the healthcare professional to exercise cultural awareness and, in particular, strong qualities in terms of equality and diversity.

Specifics in respect of personal conduct span staying within the law to meeting public expectations. Premeditated criminal acts, in particular those of a serious nature and complicity in crimes such as fraud and deception are unquestionably unacceptable failings in professional behaviour. At the other end of the spectrum, behaviours such as selfishness and disregard of the world around, for example for human suffering, cruelty to animals and the environment, would be disappointing, regrettable features of behaviour rather than a significant failing in professionalism. The public expectation of healthcare professionals, including members of the dental team and particularly dentists as team leaders, is much higher than the expectations for a 'typical person'. The wider view of society is that healthcare professionals should have higher than average levels of social responsibility and deportment. As such, society tends to be all the more critical of a healthcare professional who is guilty of antisocial or irresponsible behaviour. Each and every time a healthcare professional lets themselves down through unacceptable behaviour, they also let their profession down, eroding its standing in society.

> Public expectations for healthcare professionals are much higher than those for a 'typical person'.

142

Health and behaviour

Professional responsibilities in respect of health and behaviour require healthcare professionals to:

- seek and follow medical advice if there is any risk of passing on a serious condition to patients or colleagues
- obtain help in respect of problems that may be adversely affecting professional performance or otherwise putting patients and colleagues at risk
- cooperate fully with a procedure to investigate concerns in respect of behaviour and performance
- accept and act on concerns raised in respect of their health, behaviour or professional performance.

Duty of care

Putting patients' interests first and acting to protect them is, to many, the quintessential principle of healthcare professionalism. When a patient submits themselves to the care of a healthcare professional, including members of the dental team, they are putting great trust in the person and the associated team of healthcare providers. This trust is based on the reasonable assumption that the healthcare professionals and the people in the associate team:

- were suitably trained
- are appropriately qualified, skilled and competent
- are up to date in relevant knowledge and understanding
- will respect personal dignity and rights
- will protect the confidentiality of all personal data and disclosures
- will subscribe to the patient having the responsibility for making decisions about their healthcare priorities and what happens to them by way of treatment
- will not take actions, whether reversible or irreversible, without the patient's permission – consent
- will not suggest, let alone undertake, unnecessary treatments
- will admit to any errors or mishaps that may occur in the course of treatment and will act promptly to take the most appropriate remedial action
- will not mislead or otherwise take advantage of patients who have submitted themselves to their care.

In short: do no harm and do not abuse the patient's trust.

To help to demonstrate that the trust placed in you has been respected, and to enhance confidence in your work, it is important that the patient has the opportunity to appreciate that you have provided their treatment to the very best of your ability, using, wherever possible, evidence-based materials, techniques and procedures according to best available knowledge and understanding. In adopting this approach, it is important to remember that many oral and dental conditions can be successfully treated using more than one form of treatment. If the treatment considered most appropriate is contrary to mainstream teaching and opinion, your duty of care can still be fulfilled if the treatment is supported by a responsible body of peers, and is based on evidence sufficient to justify its application. Under such circumstances, it is prudent to advise the patient of the status of the treatment from the outset, as part of the process of obtaining consent.

Whatever the nature of treatment, duty of care may be satisfied only if the treatment falls within the range and limits of your knowledge, skills and competencies. If the treatment, let alone the diagnosis and planning of the management of the patient, falls outwith your knowledge skills and competencies, duty of care requires that you refer the patient to a colleague or other member of the dental team with the necessary advanced understanding and competencies, or, where necessary, to a specialist with advanced knowledge and expertise. If the patient decides against referral, duty of care requires that you take all possible steps to safeguard the patient, possibly through simplification of the proposed treatment. In such cases, it is particularly important to advise the patient of the possible risks and sequelae of the treatment, and to make detailed records of such advice as part of the consent procedure. Notwithstanding such measures, members of the dental team should never embark on forms of treatment that they do not understand, or that they lack the competencies to complete successfully. More importantly, if the nature of a condition is unknown, treatment should not proceed on a trial and error basis. A good rule to operate by in providing treatment, particularly irreversible forms, is: 'no diagnosis, no irreversible treatment'.

> Treatment should be based on the rule: no diagnosis, no irreversible treatment.

In investigation of allegations of a failure in respect of duty of care, an important test is whether the standard of care would be considered proper and acceptable by a reasonable body of peers. In investigation, any such allegations against a specialist in a distinct aspect of dentistry, the standard expected is normally higher than that which may be provided by a general practitioner, assuming the allegation relates to treatment within the field of that specialisation.

Child protection

Protecting children and reporting concerns in respect of child abuse and neglect are responsibilities shared by all members of society. Given that members of the dental team may observe many of the signs of child abuse and neglect, or develop concerns about the welfare of children, it is a professional responsibility to be familiar with and be able to apply procedures for child protection. A further responsibility is to ensure that children are not at risk from any member of the profession and dental procedures. Central to fulfilling these responsibilities is the ability to recognise, in particular, orofacial signs and symptoms of neglect and physical, emotional and sexual abuse in children, and knowing what to do when child abuse or neglect is suspected. Sadly, consistent themes in case of child abuse and neglect are poor communications and failures to act on suspicions, let alone evidence, of abuse or neglect. Reasons for poor communications are often related to concerns in respect of breaching patient confidentiality. If a member of the dental team has concerns about the welfare of a child, and sharing information may help to safeguard the child, consideration should be given to sharing the information even if parental consent cannot be obtained.

> There is a professional responsibility to be familiar with, and to be able to apply, procedures for child protection.

Business transactions

Three principle types of business transaction need to be considered in respect of professional behaviour and professionalism: the charging and receipt of payments for professional services; arrangements for the purchase and payment of services, equipment and consumables; and the buying, selling and running of practices.

It is often difficult for healthcare professionals to strike the right balance between professional responsibilities to their patients and the need to make a reasonable living through their practice being run as a profitable business. Serving the patients' best interests should always take precedence over profit and personal gain. If, however, this leads to a lack of profitability, the practice arrangements and the capabilities of the dental team should be the subject of critical review. Not all healthcare professionals are destined to be successful business people. Those members of the dental team who lack business acumen may well be advised to fashion their careers in a way which reduces their reliance on the business of dentistry. In addition, not all practices may be able to achieve and sustain profitability. If the profitability of a practice is threatened, the last person to bear the consequences of this must be the patient.

In all financial transactions, whether with patients, suppliers, colleagues or employees, healthcare professionals should be ethical, fair and work according to good financial practices, including the prompt settling of accounts and debts. Sharp tawdry financial practices are at best disappointing behaviour by a healthcare professional and, if of an extensive or serious nature, could well be considered a significant failure in professionalism amounting to serious professional misconduct capable of bringing the profession into disrepute. Again, the guiding principles in such matters are to treat others in the way you would wish to be treated, and, above all else, do not abuse the trust placed in you by others, in particular the trust of patients.

> Professionals must not abuse the trust placed in them by others, in particular the trust of patients.

Managerial responsibilities

Professional responsibilities for those in managerial roles include:

- setting a good example by complying with all relevant standards and guidance
- keeping up to date with skills and attitudes necessary to carry out all relevant managerial roles and responsibilities
- compliance with legal and ethical requirements, notably in relation to issues such as health and safety and equality and diversity

- maintaining honesty, integrity, fairness and openness in managing all those in the organisation or otherwise under managerial care
- delegation of only those duties which others will be able to manage
- dealing with matters expeditiously and effectively, particularly those which influence the care of patients.

Whistle blowing

Whistle blowing – bringing the behaviour or actions of a colleague to the attention of authorities – is possibly one of the most difficult and challenging aspects of professionalism. It is never easy, let alone comfortable, to report a fellow member of the dental team for inappropriate or worrisome behaviour, particularly if that person is your senior or employer. However, failure to do so may put patients at risk and, if allowed to happen, could mean that you too may be guilty of a failure in professionalism and open to a possible charge of professional misconduct. As in all relevant matters, the interests of the patient must come first.

Action needs to be taken if faced with worries and concerns, let alone evidence in respect of unacceptable professional behaviour of a colleague and that individual ignores or appears incapable of changing the behaviour in question and putting matters right. This action may save patients from suffering some form of harm and result in the person in question obtaining much-needed help. This help may be to address an underlying problem such as alcohol dependence or substance abuse, financial or personal difficulties or a health or attitudinal problem. Regrettably, there is the occasional colleague who is driven by motives other than the best interests of patients and must be removed from clinical practice to protect the public. If those closest to such individuals do not take action, irrespective of the consequences, they abnegate their responsibilities. It is unacceptable to wait until patients or others raise concerns and complaints; the delay could allow serious harm to come to patients. If needs must, the whistle needs to be blown: to do otherwise is a serious failing in professionalism. Raising concerns overrides any personal and professional loyalty.

> It is a serious failing in professionalism to avoid raising concerns: if needs require, the whistle must be blown.

Professional fulfilment

From this chapter, the reader may have formed the view that professionalism is an onerous burden, loaded with threats and few, if any, benefits. Professionalism is undoubtedly onerous, but to the vast majority of committed healthcare professionals, the burden of professionalism is far outweighed by the benefits of being a member of a healthcare profession. Being professional, through putting patients first and treating people the way you would wish to be treated, can bring great personal fulfilment. Professionalism should, therefore, be viewed positively and, wherever necessary, further developed to meet the ever-changing needs and expectations of the society that the professions exist to serve. A profession without professionalism is at best an untrustworthy trade.

Further reading

General Dental Council. Standards for Dental Professionals 2005. London: General Dental Council, 2005 Available at: http://www.gdc-uk.org/News+publications+and+events/Publications/ Guidance+documents/Standards+for+dental+professionals.htm.

Dental Protection Limited. Dental Ethics Series. London: Dental Protection Limited, 2007.

Scully C, Wilson NHF. Culturally Sensitive Oral Healthcare. [Quintessentials of Dental Practice series, Vol. 35.] London: Quintessence, 2006.

Department of Health. Child Protection and the Dental Team: An Introduction to Safeguarding Children in Dental Practice. London: The Stationery Office. Available at: www.cpdt.org.uk/www.childprotectionandthedentalteam.org.uk

Chapter 14
Confidentiality, consent and record keeping

Gail Vernon

Aim

The aim of this chapter is to outline the principles of patient confidentiality, consent and good practice in record keeping.

Outcome

Reading this chapter will give an understanding of the ways in which confidentiality, consent and record keeping are integral elements of professionalism.

Duty of confidentiality

Patients are entitled to expect that all the information the dental team learns and holds about them will remain confidential, even after their death. Information in respect of patients must be used only for the purposes for which it is given, and steps must be taken to prevent patient information from being accidentally revealed or accessed inappropriately. Patient information must be kept securely at all times.

> The duty of confidentiality applies to all members of the dental team.

Policy statement

One of the policies that a dental team should develop and apply is a policy on confidentiality. Such a policy should emphasise the importance of absolute confidentiality, and include details of the arrangements and circumstances under which patient information may be released. The policy must apply to all members of the dental team, and other members of staff who may possibly come across any information pertaining to patients. Compliance with the policy on confidentiality on a 24/7 basis should be a condition of employment for all members of the dental team.

Safeguards

To limit the risk of any breaches of confidentiality, members of the dental team should, amongst other measures:

- avoid leaving patient's clinical and other records lying around where they may be seen, for example by cleaners, visitors, tradesmen and other people who may have occasion to enter the dental premises
- ensure that patient record libraries are secure and, where necessary, supervised
- avoid taking patient's clinical records out of the dental premises, thereby precluding the risk of inadvertently leaving them in a public place or having them stolen, for example, in a briefcase from the back of a car
- be in the habit of only drawing a patient's records from the record library when they are required, and returning them to the library at the earliest possible opportunity
- keep patient's records in use out of sight of other patients and accompanying persons
- only share patient's record information with other members of the dental team on a 'need to know basis'
- exercise great care when discussing a patient; conversations are easily overheard, for example in communal areas and lifts
- be careful not to breach confidentiality when talking to patients in public areas, such as the reception area
- take steps to ensure that telephone calls to patients, or about the treatment of patients with, for example, other healthcare providers, are conducted out of earshot of others, preferably in an enclosed office
- ensure that all communications in respect of patients sent by post are mailed in sealed envelopes
- take special precautions to safeguard the security of any patient information that has been computerised
- preclude the possibility of patient information being read off a computer screen
- ensure that all processing of information pertaining to patients is conducted in accordance with relevant legislation, such as the Data Protection Act in the UK.

In considering such matters, it is important to recognise the rate at which information may be disseminated. The typical individual may share an item of new information with 15 or so people within a day. If, in turn, each of these people passes on the information to a further 15 people and so on, within two to three days more than 3000 people may be party to the information. A careless release of information, let alone gossip, particularly outwith the clinical environment, may cause significant embarrassment if not difficulty for a patient. Understandably, patients affected in this way have good reason to complain and possibly take other action in respect of the breach of confidentiality.

Releasing information

If you information about a patient has to be shared with others, this must be explained to the patient, with good reasons being given, and their permission obtained and recorded in the clinical records.

If the patient agrees to certain information being shared with someone else, it is important that the patient understands what information will be shared, the likely consequences of releasing the information and that information will be disclosed in strictest confidence only. Under other circumstances, the patient may ask you to disclose information to a third party, for example for the purpose of health insurance, or for use by legal representatives who are acting on behalf of the patient or other parties. Alternatively, other people may ask you to provide patient information, possibly including images or radiographs, for example to support teaching or research. In all cases:

- obtain the patient's consent
- make sure that the patient understands exactly what they are agreeing to and how the information will be used
- release the minimum of information necessary.

Releasing information in the public interest

From time to time it may be necessary in the public interest to share confidential information without the patient's permission. This could be information that may prevent a patient from harming themselves or others, or to identify individuals involved in serious criminal activity. In such matters, it may, given the possible consequences, be prudent to seek advice before making the disclosure. In all such circumstances, the professional should attempt to persuade the patient to disclose the relevant information themselves, or to give their permission to do so on their behalf. If this is impractical or inappropriate, consideration should be given to advising the patient of your intention to release the information; however, this may not be an option under the circumstances.

151

If a court order is received to release information without gaining permission of the patient, you the minimum information required to satisfy the order should be released.

Children and mentally compromised patients

It is a parental right to determine whether or not information in respect of a minor below 16 years of age can be released. This right, at least in the UK, terminates if and when the child achieves the understanding and intelligence to fully appreciate what is proposed. In certain circumstances, a court can override the wishes of both parents and a child in situations in which the release of information is vital to the welfare of the child. Similar arrangements apply to mentally compromised patients. If a mentally compromised patient has the understanding and intellect to fully appreciate what is proposed, decisions in respect of the release of information rests with the individual. Otherwise, the decisions rest with whoever has power of attorney for the individual.

Consent

The underpinning principle of consent is to respect patients' dignity and choices. At all times, patients must be treated with respect and allowed to exercise their rights as individuals. This requires recognition and promotion of patients' responsibility for making decisions about their bodies, priorities, care and treatment. The permission of the patient to proceed with any aspect of treatment must never be assumed; it is a general legal and ethical principle that consent is obtained prior to commencing any treatment in the care of a patient. Patients always have the right to choose whether or not to accept advice or treatment.

In a team approach to oral healthcare provision, it is important that each member of the team who treats a patient ensures that valid consent has been obtained, and that the patient consents to the various aspects of their treatment. It is not sufficient to assume that the consent obtained by the dentist, as the leader of the dental team, at the time of initial examination and treatment planning can be taken for granted. If at any time any member of the team has any uncertainties in respect of consent, the patient should be consulted to confirm their permission to proceed. This requires each member of the dental team:

- being suitably trained and qualified
- having sufficient knowledge about the proposed treatment and procedures
- understanding and being able to discuss the risks involved

If there is any doubt, the matter should be referred back to the dentist responsible for the care of the patient. At no time should a patient be rushed, let alone pushed, into a decision in respect of consent.

Forms of consent

Various forms of consent have been described (Box 14-1). Giving and getting informed consent is a process, not a one-off event, particularly given that events during treatment may lead to changes in treatment planning, risks and the clinical outcome. It is considered important that consent is based on a written treatment plan and, where indicated, an estimate of cost, particularly when complex forms of treatment are being proposed. As and when the treatment plan, and consequently the estimate of cost, may need to be changed, it is important that the patient gives informed consent to the further treatment and extra costs, or for a decision not to proceed with an element of the treatment and the accompanying risks.

In obtaining consent it is often important to:

- give the patient written, visual or other aids to understand the proposed procedures and treatment
- make special arrangements as necessary to meet special communication needs; for example, involving third parties such as a family member, close friend of the patient or interpreter, or using a hearing loop or other device
- involve all relevant members of the dental team in discussions with the patient to aid understanding of who will provide different elements of the treatment, where and when.

Above all else, the practitioner must be satisfied that the patient is fully informed and understands what is being proposed, and that the various procedures and treatments they are being asked to consent to have been fully explained. If there are concerns that the patient will be frightened or possibly put-off consenting to necessary treatment by a full and frank explanation of the proposed procedures and treatment, the challenge is to find ways to explain such matters to the patient that will not raise anxieties and doubts. It is unacceptable to 'spare' patients information that you believe will discourage them giving consent.

Voluntary decision making

To ensure that consent is valid, the relevant decisions by the patient must be made on a voluntary basis. For the decisions to be considered voluntary:

Box 14-1 **Forms of consent**

Express consent

Express consent is given when a patient volunteers orally or in writing to examination, treatment or for personal information to be processed. Express consent suffers limitations in that the patient, in volunteering their permission to proceed may not be aware of the nature, purpose and risks of the intended procedures, treatments or disclosures.

Implied consent

Implied consent occurs when, for example, a patient sits in the dental chair or opens their mouth when approached with an instrument, such as a dental mirror. Such acts do not imply that the patient fully understands what is intended, let alone the consequences or the risks. As such, implied consent is of limited value.

Specific consent

Specific consent relates to specific procedures such as the administration of conscious sedation. Such consent does not apply to related procedures; for example the treatment to be carried out on the sedated patient. Specific consent is required for patient participation in research and for the purposes of such activities as creating photographic images for teaching or publication.

Informed consent

Informed consent involves the patient understanding the nature, purpose and risks of all aspects of the proposed treatment, having the opportunity to consider all relevant information and options, to ask questions and, if necessary, to reflect on the way forward, or discuss the proposed arrangements with family and friends. For informed consent to be valid, it should be based on a fully informed balanced judgement by the patient.

- the patient must not be pressed into accepting advice or proposed arrangements
- the patient must feel that they have had opportunity to refuse, and may withdraw their consent at any time
- the patient must understand how much authority they have given the dental team.

Ability to give consent

If there is any doubt as to whether a patient is capable of giving informed consent, it is important to consider special arrangements and provisions for obtaining the consent. This may occur when dealing with mentally compromised patients, or patients who are temporarily compromised given the nature or severity of their condition. In the dental practice environment, such difficulties are typically overcome through involvement and discussions with family members or other individuals with close relationships with, or possibly responsibilities for, the patient. If in any doubt, the dentist, as the leader of the dental team, must seek advice from appropriate external agencies.

The situation regarding children is similar to that described earlier in this chapter in respect to confidentiality. It is a parental right to determine whether or not treatment is provided for a minor below 16 years of age. However, if the child achieves the understanding to appreciate what it is proposed, let alone expresses views on the planned procedures and treatment, they should be involved in the decision-making process, with their rights and opinions being respected. In the event of any uncertainties in such matters, advice should be sought.

Record keeping

Good record keeping is fundamental to good clinical practice. Patient records comprise personal information, medical histories, documentation in respect of consent, details of all relevant communications and full information in respect of all treatment provided, together with radiographs, clinical photographs, study models and all other relevant material including records of charges and payments. All elements of patient records must be meticulously maintained, treated as confidential, securely stored when not in use and seen and handled only by those who have necessity to do so.

Arrangements for patient records must comply with contemporary data protection principles; personal data must be:

- processed lawfully and fairly
- obtained only for specified and lawful purposes
- adequate, relevant and limited to what is essential
- accurate and up to date
- kept for no longer than necessary
- kept secure at all times

- processed only when necessary and, in such processes handled in accordance with relevant legislation and regulations
- only transferred or shared with consent and adequate protection.

Written records
Written records must be legible and capable of being appropriately interpreted by all those who may consult them. The use of abbreviations, notations and symbols, in particular non-standard short hand means of recording details, can lead to confusion, if not misunderstandings. Systematic, clear, comprehensive clinical records safeguard patients and provide the dental team with robust documentation if there is ever any question or criticism of the care provided. It is often important that clinical records include details of all discussions, actions and events and also matters that were not addressed or dealt with, together with reasons for such actions. If in any doubt when making written records, it is best to include rather than exclude information that may be of relevance at a later date.

Computerisation
Increasingly clinical records, including recall systems, are computerised. In adopting this approach to record keeping and handling, it is important to:

- comply with all relevant legislation and regulations, notably in respect of data protection
- ensure that the access to the computer system(s) is protected and limited to authorised personnel
- make suitable provisions for frequent, effective back-up
- make provision for suitable training, updating of systems and any necessary transfers to and between different and new systems
- be satisfied that the computerised system makes provision to record all the data you need and wish to record
- be able to link computerised records with any supportive documentation, for example signed consent forms or other materials such as study casts.

The computerisation of clinical records offers many opportunities and will undoubtedly replace most, if not all, traditional forms of records sooner rather than later. Caution must, however, be exercised in embracing computerised record systems in the interest of protecting patients, notably if the dental team has limitations in computer literacy.

Patient access to records

Patients, with certain limited exceptions, most of which do not apply to general dental practice, have rights of access to their clinical records and the right to request the correction of any inaccuracies. As a consequence, all members of the dental team should be mindful of the need to be both accurate and factual in compiling patient records. If it is considered necessary to record certain information that a patient might find embarrassing or compromising, it is good practice to advise the patient of this intention, giving reasons for the proposed actions. Inaccurate, misleading, inappropriate and unnecessary entries in clinical records can rightly and properly be cause for complaints, disciplinary actions and other measures.

Further reading and useful websites

General Dental Council:http://www.gdc-uk.org.

Chapter 15
Observing regulations
Nairn Wilson

Aim

The dental team is increasingly subject to regulation. The aim of this chapter is to outline key aspects of professional regulation and its purpose.

Outcome

This chapter enables dental team members to understand healthcare regulation better and, in particular, the regulation of dentistry.

Introduction

The principal purpose of healthcare regulation is protection of the public: putting patients' interests first and acting to protect them. Healthcare regulations and the regulation of dentistry vary internationally, ranging from being highly structured to a relatively 'light touch' approach.

> The principal purpose of healthcare regulation is protection of the public.

The various aspects of the regulation of dentistry that individually and collectively protect the public include:

- keeping up-to-date lists of practitioners and, according to national provision, other members of the dental team entitled to provide and otherwise be involved in the provision of oral healthcare
- setting high standards of dental practice and conduct
- maintaining high standards of dental education
- requiring members of the dental team to be lifelong learners through participation in continuing professional development (CPD)
- taking action if there is any doubt about the conduct or competency of any registered dental healthcare professional.

159

Registration of a dental healthcare professional is not simply an administrative process. Registration typically demonstrates that the individual has satisfied demanding standards and is maintaining and updating their skills and knowledge through lifelong learning and, in time, revalidation.

> Registration demonstrates that an individual has satisfied demanding standards and is maintaining and updating skills and knowledge.

The General Dental Council – the sole, competent, regulatory authority for dentistry in the UK – sets out six key principles to define the modern dental healthcare professional. These principles are:

- putting patients' interests first and acting to protect them
- respecting patients' dignity and choices
- protecting the confidentiality of patients' information
- cooperating with other members of the dental team and other healthcare colleagues in the interests of patients
- maintaining professional knowledge and competence
- being trustworthy.

Regulation, although demanding, underpins public confidence and the standing of the profession. To satisfy the ever-increasing expectations of the public, healthcare regulation has had to become more open, transparent, accountable and, most importantly, demanding of dental healthcare professionals. This development is set to continue, as society becomes more questioning and demanding of those accorded the privilege and status of being healthcare professionals.

> Regulation forms the basis for public confidence and the standing of the profession.

Indemnity

An important aspect of the regulatory requirement laid on healthcare professionals is the need to be indemnified. Certain employers, such as the NHS in the UK, provide indemnity to protect the patient. Full (comprehensive) professional indemnity is, however, strongly recommended to safeguard both the patient and the professional standing of the dental clinician. In a society that is increasingly litigious, the best available professional indemnity is strongly recommended.

> The professional is strongly recommended to have full (comprehensive) professional indemnity.

Conclusions

The regulation of dentistry is primarily aimed at protecting the public. Although demanding, the regulation of dentistry is important to the present and future standing of the profession and the trust placed in it by the public. The regulation of dentistry is increasing open transparent and accountable to help to reinforce the emphasis on the protection of the public.

Further reading and useful websites

General Dental Council:http://www.gdc-uk.org.

Chapter 16
Keeping up to date

Gail Vernon

Aim

The aim of this chapter is to outline the importance of continuing professional development (CPD), the aspects of clinical practice which should receive special attention in CPD, and possible arrangements for planning, accessing and recording CPD activities.

Outcome

Having read this chapter, members of the dental team should better understand the need for CPD, and be able to use CPD activities to keep up to date, both individually and collectively.

Introduction

The rate of introduction of new technologies, procedures and treatment in dentistry is set to increase. If innovations in clinical practice since the mid to late 1990s have been impressive, the prediction is that these will pale into insignificance given anticipated, developments, let alone unexpected developments, in the next 10 to 15 years. Such prospects make the future of dentistry exciting and dynamic, but it emphasises the increasing importance of CPD for all members of the dental team. It has long been recognised that members of the dental team need to be lifelong learners to keep up to date – students for life – both to learn new things and to maintain essential skills and knowledge. Indeed, an increasing number of licensing and regulatory dental bodies around the world require dental personnel to be actively engaged in CPD as part of relicensing requirements. Healthcare CPD is widely accepted to be important for the protection of patients and for further development of the healthcare professions, including dentistry. In dentistry, certain aspects of CPD are increasingly viewed as compulsory. For example, the General Dental Council in the UK requires, in addition to CPD relevant to specific areas of practice, CPD in the so-called core subjects: medical emergencies, disinfection and decontamination, radiography and radiation protection. Members of the dental team participating in postgraduate or postqualification training may need to check with their licensing or regulatory body as to whether their studies count towards CPD requirements.

> All members of the dental team should be lifelong learners.

Notwithstanding the requirements of licensing and regulatory bodies, it should be considered a professional responsibility to maintain essential skills and knowledge and to keep abreast of developments in clinical practice to best serve the needs of patients. Furthermore, keeping up to date and being familiar with developments in clinical practice can greatly add to professional fulfilment. For example, it should be very rewarding to the dental team to be able to restore an edentulous gap efficiently and effectively using implant therapy where, previously, it would have been necessary to resort to a less-satisfactory or more interventional means of achieving a satisfactory clinical outcome.

Forms of continuing professional development

There are many forms of CPD, both specific and general. For CPD to be recognised for the purpose of relicensing or similar procedures (verifiable) by licensing and regulatory bodies, various requirements needs to be satisfied. These requirements typically include:

- the activity needs to have clear aims, objectives and anticipated outcomes
- the activity needs to be quality controlled, with participants having the opportunity, possibly the requirement, to provide feedback on the strengths and weaknesses of the activity
- documentary evidence of attendance and participation in the activity.

In addition to traditional forms of CPD such as attending lectures, courses, conferences, hands-on programmes, books and other publications, there are many new forms of CPD, for example:

- journal article CPD questionnaires and tests
- web-based distance and flexible, self-directed CPD
- interactive CPD activities through various websites
- television, video, CD ROM and audio-based programme materials.

Notwithstanding the expanding range of opportunities and media for CPD, many members of the dental team continue to have a strong preference for activities involving face-to-face interactions and meeting up with professional colleagues. Consequently, it is anticipated that traditional activities such as national association and specialist society meetings and conferences will continue to have a future. At the same time, the needs of dental teams working in remote or atypical circumstances will increasingly be met through the use of new technologies.

It is suggested that forms of verifiable CPD should be supplemented by more general forms of CPD including:

- purchasing and reading journals and books
- participation in local study clubs
- gleaning new information in respect of products and devices from company representatives, literature and websites
- involvement in professional bodies and societies.

Record keeping: portfolios

Even if this were not a requirement of licensing and regulatory bodies, it is good practice to keep detailed records of CPD activities, ideally in the form of a personal development portfolio, including reflection on CPD activities and identifying areas of weaknesses and future CPD needs. Through the use of such a portfolio, members of the dental team may be best placed to manage their individual and collective CPD requirements. If such a portfolio is not used, it is all too easy to indulge in CPD in the 'comfort zone' rather than meeting needs in more challenging and demanding areas.

Whatever records of CPD activity are kept, it is important that these include any information necessary for purposes of auditing. In addition to personal details, key information to record includes:

- the date, nature and title of the activity
- the aims, objectives and anticipated outcomes
- the venue or media
- details of the provider
- the number of hours spent on the activity
- reflections on the value and benefits of the activity.

Conclusions

All healthcare professionals need to use CPD for both the requirements of their professional organisations and to keep up to date with the rapid changes in their field. The checklist below is a suggested way to organise CPD.

- Plan how to meet necessary and required CPD in terms of both hours completed and topics covered. Be mindful that a specified amount of CPD should be verifiable rather than just general.
- Choose a recording format that is easy to use and keeps everything together. This may be a CPD portfolio provided by the professional association or a recording form provided by the licensing or regulatory body.
- In addition to certificates of attendance, it may be useful to retain programmes of events. This is a useful way of supporting records and recalling speakers, topics and time spent on different aspects of clinical practice.
- When deciding whether to carry out general CPD activities, considering if it will contribute to your CPD.
- If spending time away and, in particular, paying for verifiable CPD, check that the educational criteria laid down by the regulatory body will be satisfied and ensure that there is documentary evidence of your participation, including the number of hours of activity.
- Review activities on a regular basis to ensure that minimum requirements will be met. Avoid having to do large amounts of CPD just ahead of some deadline: CPD is most beneficial if organized on an ongoing basis.
- Finally, do not hesitate to seek assistance from your professional association or licensing/regulatory body if advice is needed.

Further sources of information

General Dental Council:http://www.gdc-uk.org.

Health Professions Council. Your Guide to our Standards for Continuing Professional Development. London: Health Professions Council, 2005.

Index

Quintessentials of Dental Practice Series

in 44 volumes

Editor-in-Chief: Professor Nairn H F Wilson

The Quintessentials of Dental Practice Series covers basic principles and key issues in all aspects of modern dental medicine. Each book can be read as a stand-alone volume or in conjunction with other books in the series.

Clinical Practice, Editor: Nairn Wilson

Culturally Sensitive Oral Healthcare
Dental Erosion
Special Care Dentistry
Evidence-based Dentistry
Infection Control for the Dental Team

Oral Surgery and Oral Medicine, Editor: John G Meechan

Practical Dental Local Anaesthesia
Practical Oral Medicine
Practical Conscious Sedation
Minor Oral Surgery in Dental Practice

Imaging, Editor: Keith Horner

Interpreting Dental Radiographs
Panoramic Radiology
21st Century Dental Imaging

Periodontology, Editor: Iain L C Chapple

Understanding Periodontal Diseases: Assessment and
    Diagnostic Procedures in Practice
Decision-Making for the Periodontal Team
Successful Periodontal Therapy: A Non-Surgical Approach
Periodontal Management of Children, Adolescents and
    Young Adults
Periodontal Medicine: A Window on the Body
Contemporary Periodontal Surgery: An Illustrated Guide
    to the Art Behind the Science

Endodontics, Editor: John M Whitworth

    Rational Root Canal Treatment in Practice
    Managing Endodontic Failure in Practice
    Adhesive Restoration of Endodontically Treated Teeth

Prosthodontics, Editor: P Finbarr Allen

    Teeth for Life for Older Adults
    Complete Dentures – from Planning to Problem Solving
    Removable Partial Dentures
    Fixed Prosthodontics in Dental Practice
    Applied Occlusion
    Orofacial Pain: A Guide for General Practitioners

Operative Dentistry, Editor: Paul A Brunton

    Decision-Making in Operative Dentistry
    Aesthetic Dentistry
    Communicating in Dental Practice
    Indirect Restorations
    Dental Bleaching
    Dental Materials in Operative Dentistry
    Successful Posterior Composites

Paediatric Dentistry/Orthodontics, Editor: Marie Therese Hosey

    Child Taming: How to Manage Children in Dental Practice
    Paediatric Cariology
    Treatment Planning for the Developing Dentition
    Managing Dental Trauma in Practice

General Dentistry and Practice Management, Editor: Raj Rattan

    The Business of Dentistry
    Risk Management in General Dental Practice
    Quality Matters: From Clinical Care to Customer Service

Dental Team, Editor: Mabel Slater

    Dental Team Companion

Implantology, Editor: Lloyd J Searson

    Implantology in General Dental Practice

Quintessence Publishing Co. Ltd., London

Dental team companion.